SLEEP YOUR FAT AWAY

SLEEP YOUR FAT AWAY

TRAIN YOUR BRAIN TO LOSE WEIGHT EFFORTLESSLY

**JOY MARTINA Ph.D. AND
ROY MARTINA M.D.**
#1 HOLISTIC THOUGHT LEADERS

New York

SLEEP YOUR FAT AWAY
TRAIN YOUR BRAIN TO LOSE WEIGHT EFFORTLESSLY

© 2015 **JOY MARTINA Ph.D. AND ROY MARTINA M.D.**.

Published in New York, New York, by Morgan James Publishing. Morgan James and The Entrepreneurial Publisher are trademarks of Morgan James, LLC.
www.MorganJamesPublishing.com

The Morgan James Speakers Group can bring authors to your live event. For more information or to book an event visit The Morgan James Speakers Group at www.TheMorganJamesSpeakersGroup.com.

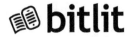

A **free** eBook edition is available with the purchase of this print book.

CLEARLY PRINT YOUR NAME ABOVE IN UPPER CASE

Instructions to claim your free eBook edition:
1. Download the BitLit app for Android or iOS
2. Write your name in **UPPER CASE** on the line
3. Use the BitLit app to submit a photo
4. Download your eBook to any device

ISBN 978-1-63047-460-7 paperback
ISBN 978-1-63047-461-4 eBook
Library of Congress Control Number:
2014917921

Cover Design by:
Chris Treccani
www.3dogdesign.net

Interior Design by:
Bonnie Bushman
bonnie@caboodlegraphics.com

In an effort to support local communities and raise awareness and funds, Morgan James Publishing donates a percentage of all book sales for the life of each book to Habitat for Humanity Peninsula and Greater Williamsburg.

Get involved today, visit
www.MorganJamesBuilds.com

Habitat
for Humanity®
Peninsula and
Greater Williamsburg
Building Partner

Disclaimer

Sleep Your Fat Away offers general information about losing weight using special types of exercises, visualizations, lifestyle changes and behaviors, which are commonly believed to support a healthy weight loss. However, each person is unique and the information included in this book may not be appropriate for your specific health or mental situation. The Sleep Your Fat Away Program does not give medical advice or opinions on medical conditions, treatments, or cures; and you should not rely upon anything in the Sleep Your Fat Away Program materials as a preventive, cure, or treatment for any purposes. If you have any medical condition or doubts about this program consult a licensed health professional. The Sleep Your Fat Away Program is designed to teach you how to apply mental techniques and healthy eating habits to kick start the weight loss you desire. Any information in The Sleep Your Fat Away Program or downloadable audio-package that appears in the form of an opinion, recommendation, preventive, cure or treatment should NOT be taken as conventional medical or other advice even if it may appear to you as such. The authors strongly recommend that you check with a licensed physician, who is familiar with the details of your particular situation before you begin using The Sleep Your Fat Away Program or The Sleep Your Fat Away Program downloadable materials.

No warranties: The Sleep Your Fat Away program provides the system and system materials "as is" without warranty of any kind, either expressed or implied, including, but not limited to, the implied warranties of merchantability, health, healing or weight loss.

Anti-virus: The authors do not warrant that the Sleep Your Fat Away website will operate error-free or that its system website and its server are free of computer viruses or other harmful mechanisms. If your use of the Sleep Your Fat Away website or Sleep Your Fat Away materials results in the need for servicing or replacing equipment or data, the authors and associates are not responsible for those costs.

Your health and weight is your responsibility, always: Your health is your responsibility and your responsibility only. Your use of The Sleep Your Fat Away Program is your choice and will be at your own risk. The Sleep Your Fat Away Program materials are not intended to offer you all information about maintaining a healthy slim body, mind, and soul. There are many options and alternative courses of action that may be equally or more beneficial to you. Exploring all of the options and alternatives is your responsibility. The Sleep Your Fat Away Program materials include descriptions and demonstrations of certain exercises, guided meditations and use of audio programs. You are responsible, should you decide to incorporate them into your daily routine. Descriptions of, or references to, products or publications do not imply endorsement of that product or publication.

Limitation of Liability: The authors and its publisher, subsidiary and affiliated companies and their respective directors, shareholders, officers, employees, advisors, agents, licensors, and other contributors will not be liable for any injury, harm or death you or others may suffer as a result of the use or attempted use of The Sleep Your Fat Away Program or any materials in this book or accompanying audio programs and materials, whether or not such use is in accordance with all The Sleep Your Fat Away instructions or other directions. The authors and their associates will not be liable for any indirect, consequential, special, incidental or punitive damages related to The Sleep Your Fat Away Program materials or any errors or omissions related thereto. The Sleep Your Fat Away Program maximum liability for any claim based upon this program or program materials is limited to the retail price of The Sleep Your Fat Away Program as of the date of publication of the version or edition. Because some states and countries do not allow the exclusion or limitation of liability for consequential or incidental damages, the above limitation may not apply to you.

Dedication

We dedicate this book to all the children of this world who are suffering either from malnutrition by our modern processed foods or due to the lack of sufficient food.

Our hearts go out to them and we pledge that part of the profits of The Sleep Your Fat Away Program will be donated to causes related to helping our young ones have a better healthier and happier life!

Table of Contents

Acknowledgements

We thank our parents for their endless support and love. We appreciate your dedication to raising us the way you did and thank you for motivating us to look after our health and well being, make informed choices and strive for the best.

We give thanks to our children: Sunray, Joey, Jacob, George, and Grace for being in our lives and holding the mirror to us. We love you more than you will ever know.

We also want to acknowledge Sheila Granger for inspiring us to take the Virtual Gastric Band to a whole new level!

About the Authors

Joy & Roy Martina

Sleep Your Fat Away is the result of years of researching, testing and improving upon techniques designed to train your brain to respond in a way similar to naturally slim people. The story begins with Roy; he was diagnosed at an early age with brain damage because of asphyxia at birth. Asphyxia means lack of oxygen. He came out quite blue and had to be resuscitated. He spent a few days recovering in isolation.

Born fat

Roy was a truly fat baby; actually he was the heaviest baby in the hospital. His struggle to take back control of his life began at an early age. At the age of six, Roy was aggressive, angry, and regularly reprimanded for fighting with other kids, who were teasing (bullying) him.

Sports as a way to battle fat

At the age of six, he was, on the advice of a psychotherapist, sent to judo (martial arts) as a way of anger management. This worked very well and Roy blossomed under the guidance of his sensei (teacher), who was like a mentor to him. He learned how to respect others, deal with his anger issues, and grow up a happier kid.

There were, however, two areas where he was not succeeding: loosing his baby-fat and his lack of focus. He was hyperactive, had low self-esteem, started dieting at the age of ten, and exercised 2-3 hours daily. This worked for his weight as he was gradually getting slimmer and start to excel as an athlete and won over four hundred competitions in martial arts, table tennis, tennis, swimming and karate.

Discovering sleep programming

At the age of 11, Roy still had problems keeping his focus in class. He decided to do an experiment and in 1964 started recording all the class materials he had to study on a tape whilst doing his homework. At that time the tape recorders had these big reels of tape and you could easily record for many hours at a time. During the night he would put on headphones and go to sleep. The results were astonishing; he had instant and total recall of all the facts he had put on tape. The subject did not matter: it could be math, geography, history, books, languages; everything he put on tape he immediately had access to at any given time. This catapulted him to the best in class. His measured IQ was at the level of a so-called genius. He graduated from his school as the best student they had ever had; some of those records have not even been broken today (2014). Roy also developed an interest in psychology and personal development at the age of 13 and started adding positive suggestions for other areas of his life to his recordings. He was mainly interested in sports and the sleep programming helped him to have more motivation, stamina, improve his tennis, martial arts, and all the other sports he was competing in. He was the first all round student to excel in sports, languages, math, he graduated as the best in class (cum laude) and he was champion in tennis, judo and table tennis.

College and sleep programming

Roy went to study medicine and applied the sleep program to his medical studies and was one of the youngest students to graduate at the age of 22 cum laude in the Netherlands. He also became European judo champion, karate champion, kick box champion and was undefeated in more than 150 fights. All these successes were due to his use of the sleep-programming concept.

Holistic medicine and sleep programming

After his medical studies he continued his studies in natural medicine and became a holistic doctor using acupuncture, homeopathy, herbs, supplements and nutrition to help over 100,000 patients regain their health from chronic disease.

He also helped people to lose weight and keep it off for years.

In 2012 Joy and Roy discovered a new technique via hypnosis and decided to test it out with the concept of sleep programming. It worked on hundred's of clients in Europe. A new way to help people lose weight and keep it off was born. Roy tested this on himself and lost over 40 pounds.

A little bit more about Joy & Roy

We encourage and assist you in training your brain, opening your heart, and nurturing your soul. We have dedicated our lives to assisting people transform their lives by giving them practical tools to help themselves. We believe in your power to live your potential even if you have given up. We know that you can lose weight in your sleep and become a naturally slim person!

We are

- Health food worshippers (we *love* eating good food and enjoying life!)
- Work out lovers
- And never go to bed angry.

We know what it's like to

- Be addicted to sugar

- Hate your body
- Feel bad about yourself because you've failed yet another diet
- Suffer cravings and
- Be overweight.

We've been there, we've done that, and we won the battle. Today we are healthy, happy, and slim and <u>you can do the same</u>.

We are here to help you.

Joy Martina is a Rapid Change Coach, the creator of the Christallin Method Training, Master Hypnotist and Trainer of Trainers. She is passionate about helping people get back into their power. She adores showing people the way out of their stuck states and inspiring them to enjoy life again.

- Her approach is based on her ability to connect to the subconscious mind and get directly to the cause of the problems: Digging out the concealed information that is even hidden from the clients themselves and solving the issues right where they started.
- She is also a Strategic Business Consultant helping Corporations make strategic choices that enhance their success and profitability.
- She is the co-author of 6 books. She leads the ICON (International Christallin Oracles Network) a dedicated group of Oracles that continues training and doing research about the future.

Joy used to eat insane amounts of chocolate without feeling nauseated. There were times when there was NO day without chocolate. She suffered from mood swings, irritability, and fatigue – all because of highly volatile blood sugar levels caused by an excess intake of sugar. Today she has given up on sugar and processed foods completely and is healthier, happier, and more vital than ever before. Thanks to the Sleep Your Fat Away Program she was able to banish cravings for good and is still astounded at how painless that was!

Roy Martina is a world renowned Holistic Medical Doctor, the no #1 Holistic Thought Leader of Europe, best selling author, the creator of the Omega Healing Method and teaches with Joy world-wide on many different subjects.

- He has written over 70 books, many have been translated into more than 10 languages. One of his best sellers is Emotional Balance (Hay House). You can find this book on amazon.com.
- Roy is passionate about health, longevity, and fitness and is integrating all that he learns into the Omega method.
- He has been training over 250,000 people including doctors, professors, therapists, coaches, and managers worldwide for over 25 years.

Roy has a life long history in dieting. As a fanatic researcher in all health related matters he would try almost every diet and promising supplement on this planet. He was a master at yo-yo dieting and only due to his love for exercise was he able to keep his weight from skyrocketing. Sleep Your Fat Away literally saved his life from living a constant battle with his weight. Roy lost 40 pounds in 6 months and has kept his ideal weight since. No battle, no feeling of deprivation but lots of energy instead!

Do you want to know how to Sleep Your Fat Away?

Are you ready to become a naturally slim person? Then read at least up until chapter 8 and find out how! You will not regret it – we promise!

If you are not an avid reader or are keen to get results even before finishing the book, you can start right away! Just read the introduction and get on your way to a healthy, happy slim you!

Preface:

The Secret Behind the Power of the Mind
and How You Can Take Control of Your Life

Body—Spirit Essence—Mind

When you are born into this world, you are given a sophisticated self-regulating biological organism (a **body**), which is given life by your **spirit** essence (whatever that is) and you have a bio-computer system in your brain, which we call **mind**.

Training your brain (mind)

Your mind is programmed by the environment in order for you to adapt to whatever challenges you are facing in that environment. So primitive farming communities would teach their children to farm and hunters will teach their offspring how to hunt. In this modern world we have 3 educational systems working simultaneously: your parents (your primary role models), your teachers and peers (your secondary role models or educators) and the media (TV, movies and other media). The media power has become more and more digital, and we are being exposed to this digital reality at an increasingly younger age.

These 3 systems create what is called your Mental Conditioning and the way you react and behave in our 3-dimensional world.

Your self-image is created in your first 7 years

Your parents, peers, environment, religion, media, and the books you read, etc. condition your behavioral patterns, thinking process and finally create your self-image!

How you express yourself is not who you are but who you believe you are. Your self-image is not you; it is a false construction in your mind based on your life-experience, the instilled beliefs and the way you give meaning to your experiences.

Digital reality: the wrong way to train your brain

New technology has brought us many new possibilities and in many ways makes our life easier and faster. Yet it also entails a huge danger for us and even more so for the young ones. It is fascinating to study how this really works and how we are being conditioned to respond to it. The ramifications are far stretching! The quicksand of technology is rewiring our brains and our hearts. Too much, too soon often results in a shorter attention span (the whole world is becoming more hyper active and reactive), less exercise, superficial relationships, loss of self control and sustained thought, hearing loss (from the high volumes of headphones), fried brain cells from exposure to heat and infrared from cellphones held close to the head, social isolation (with the prevalence of social media, the rate of younger people acquiring drivers licenses is going down), sleep disorders, plagiarism, disrupted hormones, shallowness, fear of silence and obesity in children is rising at a speed never seen before in history.

As a consequence the late onset diabetes type 2, formerly only seen in ages of 40 and up, is rising in overweight teenagers. High-density stimulation emboldens hurtful speech and aggressive behavior (bullying) off line and online while decreasing compassion, empathy and the ability to recognize facial expressions and voice tones.

Prevention is the mother of all cures

As a parent you have to take control. Don't expose infants and toddlers to too much technology and from ages three to six limit exposure times to less than 2 hours a day. It's best to increase this time slowly and keep it to a minimum.

Balance screen usage with plenty of outside activities, exercise, fresh air, walks in nature, friendships, conversation, household chores, pet care, gardening and learning how to cook, drawing, music etc.

It is, of course, more work but the benefits will last a lifetime. Each child that is saved from becoming addicted to useless games that promote aggression and destruction is a blessing. It is not too late to prevent or lessen the effects the over consumption of technology is having on the mental health of a generation. And remember: You don't have to do this on your own. Conscious parenting is not about the **<u>amount</u>** of time you spend with your kids. It's about the **<u>quality</u>** of time you spend with them. Make every hour you spend with your children count and make use of qualified instructors, teachers, mentors and helpers to guide and entertain your kids in empowering and positive ways if you don't have enough time to do so yourself.

Digital technology: Use it to train your child's brains (...and your own!)

We can also use technology to our advantage. Our daughter, Grace, is 4 years old and she also benefits already from sleep programming. We have several audio sessions that she listens to; one is especially made for kids and takes them on a magical journey to a world where they learn about self-esteem, self-respect, and helping out. She listens to that in German and English. She loves choosing the program she wants to listen too and another favorite is one boosting her self-healing powers, which is full of positive suggestions. We have seen her blossom and become a much happier and more loving, open person since she started to listen to positive messages whilst sleeping. She is less fearful and far more confident. She loves the sleep programs so much that she kicks up quite a fuss when we forget to take them with us when travelling. Her pre-school now also plays them during nap-hour and the kids love their "bedtime stories"!

Our teenagers also have their own sleep programs to listen to and their grades improved greatly since they started to train their brains at night. We ourselves also listen to sleep programming every night, and get to choose from several subjects: loving relationships, eliminating sabotage, promoting success and wealth, health and self-worth. We are fanatic about the making the most of the limitless possibilities and are developing new programs, which we want to make accessible to millions, so they can also start their process of never ending improvement of life-quality.

Most suffering is self-inflicted (karma)

Karma is a sometimes an overly used word and often put in the box of "woo-woo spirituality". But karma is not a mystery: simply put it is "the consequences of your choices." Every choice you make has a consequence. Ignorance will present you with limitations of your options. Going against your body's intelligence will result in suffering long term and sometimes already short term. Most so-called aging-related diseases are the result of wrong choices. Dementia for instance is caused by plaques in the brain circulation and can be prevented if one knows what to do. Longevity is only partially due to genetic disposition, the rest depends upon knowing what to do; losing weight is part of that!

By not understanding how to take control of your body and mind, you will exponentially increase the probability of suffering discomfort, shortening your genetic potential of longevity and attracting unnecessary negative situations.

This can also be called **mental-physical karma** and is the result of the accumulative consequences of your lifestyle.

Our promise

With this book and the mind program we created: "Sleep Your Fat Away," you have the tools to change how you relate to your body, your weight, your food and eating habits. You can become slim and stay slim for life!

You will be able to lengthen your life span, become, and stay slim, healthy, and happy. Using the power of your mind, you can change your eating habits, work on the causal effects of being overweight, and finally enjoy exercising like never before. It is all up to you. We will provide you with tools that are simple, powerful, and easy to use.

There are only 3 steps to take:

- Read this book to make sure you understand all the principles
- Follow the guidelines
- Get the program and <u>start losing weight in your sleep</u>

We know that if you do, you will be successful. Without diets, pills, and without having to kill yourself with aerobic exercises.

Joy & Roy Martina

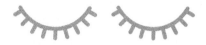

Introduction

The Law of Insanity:

Why Diets, Pills, Exercise, and Willpower are Setting You Up for Failure

E instein said: "The law of insanity is trying the same thing over and over again and expecting a different outcome!"

Our mothers are experts in dieting

Roy often jokingly says in workshops: "My mother has lost more weight than an adult elephant. Sadly, she gained it all back again!"

Both our mothers have tried out over 40 different diets and are walking encyclopedias on diets and the differences.

Roy's mum went to Weight-Watchers for years and that was the only system that kept her on a path to lose weight. But as soon as she stopped going to the meetings, the yo-yo effect came back swinging in full force.

Joy's Mom

As long as I can remember, my mother was on a diet. A vivid memory of mine is that at family dinners, we would all have our plates full of food except for Mummy. All she would be eating was half a grapefruit. I grew up seeing my beautiful mother struggle with her weight. She would deprive herself for some time, suffer while doing so, and then fall back into her old habits as soon as willpower failed her. Her excess weight was directly connected to a decreasing level of self-confidence. As much as she detested being overweight, she became increasingly sensitive to any comments (or even looks) related to her figure and would not accept any form of assistance. It was heart breaking as a daughter to see this amazing woman being seemingly beaten by the weight game and the health issues that came with the excess fat – and not be able to do anything for her. When I was finally able and allowed to help, it was a game changer. At last my beloved Mum was able to break the destructive patterns of over-eating and be the healthy, slim and happy lady she is today. And you can imagine how thrilled I was, when she sent us her testimonial:

"I am an expert on diets. Throughout my wonderful and exciting life there is no diet worth writing about that I haven't tried. I have counted calories, joules, fat units, carbohydrates, and fiber. I have separated carbohydrates from protein, I have eaten fat with protein, I have gone totally vegetarian, and enjoyed a Mediterranean diet. You name it and I have tried it. My weight has yo-yoed more than a work out on a trampoline and over the years I must have lost more than the weight of a baby elephant, and gained it all back again. Does this sound familiar?

The "Sleep Your Fat Away" program is the only program that has shown me that I can get and maintain a body that I am proud of. Initially I was skeptical of the program but as the weeks turned into months I thoroughly enjoyed losing weight, with no effort at all. Not only did those awful hunger pains disappeared but I had so much more energy. I even started running again, and enjoyed it. I found that I automatically chose to eat more vegetables and fruit, and no longer craved sweets and chocolates.

My weight loss was steady and constant; at no time did I feel that I was "on a diet." The Sleep Your Fat Away program has become a way of life and I feel amazing."

Sylvia: Health Coach in Italy

This story is not only our mother's story. We have heard it over and over again from many of my clients who have tried a myriad of diets and pills. A typical story is of Sylvia from Italy, who came to our workshop to learn the technique Sleep Your Fat Away. We have known her for a few years and had seen that she would be much happier as a coach if she could shed some weight. Sylvia was 38 years old and her story goes like this:

During my second pregnancy (I was 28 years old) I got cravings for sweets and started indulging in them on a daily basis. In Italy we believe that depriving yourself during pregnancy is depriving the baby. So you have the excuse to indulge in your cravings without guilt and that is exactly what I did. At the end of my pregnancy I had ballooned to an extra 15 kilos (33 pounds) of fat, but during breastfeeding I got a craving for cheese and again I indulged in big amounts of cheese and you know how we Italians love our cheese.

In the end she was 42 pounds over her normal weight. She had done the "Fit for Life", Atkins diet, Paleo-diet, and at least 10 more to no avail, the story was always the same: in the beginning everything worked perfectly and she would lose weight rapidly. But after 3-4 weeks, her willpower would lessen and she would start binging, feeling guilty and like a loser and soon she would give up. She had also tried hypnosis, acupuncture, and exercise but did not manage to keep any weight lost off. On the contrary: By now she was 58 pounds above her normal weight! Life had become difficult for her because she felt as a coach that she had failed and her business was also no longer the thriving practice she had in the beginning. For her, the most painful part of the story (she was crying) was when she had to admit defeat. She felt she was a lost case, unattractive and a bad mother because she couldn't be the good role model she wanted to be for her two kids. She said that food helped her eat her pain away!

She came to the workshop because she believed in our methods as she was trained by us to be a Health Coach. She said: "I am so happy that you finally decided to tackle this problem! If it works for me I can help the hundred's of people I know, who are suffering from the same problem and I will be back on track to being who I really am!

The band that changed our future

Going back to our mothers, the gastric band was a changing point in their lives – as it was for us. We discovered that the trick was to teach people to start listening to their bodies again. (See chapter 6 Shrink your Stomach and Lose Weight Effortlessly with the Virtual Gastric Band)

The gastric band forces you to eat less and feel satisfied sooner, so we decided to find a way of applying that concept to our practice without the surgery. We learnt from our mothers who, like Sylvia, were experts on dieting. They didn't need more knowledge about <u>what</u> to eat, they needed a strategy that helped them reconnect to their body's intelligence and learn <u>how</u> to eat.

Theory is overrated.

If you have done more than 4-5 diets you are an expert on diets and you know all you need to know of what does not work.

Each book you read tackles another aspect or theory of diet. One fad follows the next. They all work in some way but the question is:

Why don't they work for everybody?

And why don't you get the consistent effects that last a lifetime?

Every day millions of people go on a low calorie or a low carbohydrate or a fat-free diet; they try the sugar free diet, the boost your metabolism diet, the caveman diet… you name it they've tried it.

We have seen Dr. Atkins and the South Beach diet come and go.

We have had "Fit for life": on how to combine foods to lose weight and stay fit. We had the Blood type diet, the "Metabolic diet," and low fat diets, the Weight Watchers, etc.

Most of you have tried out many diets and always fall in the same pattern: you lose some weight and over time gain it back again.

Dieting by starving or depriving yourself has so far only helped many people feel miserable and enhanced their daily struggle with food. We will talk later about the three triggers of the subconscious mind that will sound an alarm bell in your mind and cause havoc to any diet you will undertake. They are known as the 3 D's: Diet, Deprivation, and Discipline (will power). The D-words are red flags for your subconscious mind and will trigger a myriad of sabotage mechanisms to bring you back to sanity!

Maybe you are one of these admirable people who have spent a lot of time and money on various diets and have struggled with will power for many years.

Sleep your weight off? Seriously? You must be kidding me!

Now you hear about a weight loss program that is NOT a diet, it's not about taking pills or having to exercise and you can lose weight in your sleep? And you think: this sounds too good to be true!

We hear that all the time and people often will not even hear us out because they think we are insane, yet the whole system is based on the science of how the brains work and how they influence your metabolism, so bear with us and we will show you that this is not a myth or fad. You CAN lose weight in your sleep and become a naturally slim person!

All of the above theories and diets do work in theory and they are based on scientific facts.

But in the end it is not about the theory. It is about the human factor, the person having to stick to the theory.

7 points we would like to see in an effective weight-loss program:

1. Did it change your life style and eating habits?
2. Are you happier and more emotionally stable as the result?
3. Is it healthy for your body?
4. Is it sustainable? Can you do it the rest of your life?
5. Is it easy, joyous, and gracious or do you feel you are being deprived?
6. Do you need willpower to do it or are you on automatic pilot?
7. Is it effective? Are you losing weight steadily, even when you have little fall backs?

Our program contains these 7 factors. We have created a system of brain training, which makes weight loss easy and effective, with over 90% proven long-lasting results.

Are you ready to understand that it is not about dieting but about changing the way you think about food and yourself? We will give you the theory you need to know:

- How to increase your fat burning metabolism during the night so you can relax around food.
- Why it takes nothing else than listening to some audio programming while you sleep and or during the daytime to change how you deal with food for the rest of your life.
- How we have helped thousands of people all over the world change their life, finally lose weight and keep it off permanently.
- How you can break the cycle of millions of people worldwide who are getting fatter each year and who are experiencing the disastrous effects being overweight has on their health.

It does not matter if you need to lose 5 or 50 or 100 pounds:

You can win this battle, succeed in lowering your fat percentage, and <u>become a naturally slim person for life</u>!

Sylvia: Health Coach in Italy, continued

Sylvia followed the 3-day workshop for Practitioners in Germany and what was interesting that during the workshop she lost already 2 pounds! Why? Because as practitioners they had to practice on each other and the virtual gastric band was installed on the second day and on the 3rd day we worked on creating aversion on the foods that were addictive and attraction on healthy foods. Just by changing how she ate (you will learn that in this book) and having her sessions (you can get those on <u>www.sleepyourfataway.com</u>) she started to shed the pounds gradually and effortlessly. After 4 weeks she wrote us the following email: "Dear Joy and Roy, you have saved my emotional health, my marriage and my coaching practice! I feel now so good about myself and new clients are calling every day and I have an insane amount of word of mouth referrals and that because I feel alive again and have more energy than when I was 23 years old. The best part is that I now have a group of women I am coaching to lose weight and they are all doing well! Thank you, thank you, thank you!

Can I do this by myself?

If you mean: Can you buy the program and do it by yourself? Yes! That's the plan! We created a program which is so easy to follow that people can follow it in their own pace and get the results without needing extra help. We believe in empowering people to help themselves.

An alternative is to see a trained Sleep Your Fat Away Expert and work with him/her in private sessions; this can also be done by Skype. That has the advantage of being able to talk about what makes you unique, what your personal struggles with weight loss are and they can address that. In our program we have covered issues that we have come across in our mutual 45 years of practice. That is why this program is so effective. In our sleep program we have covered all corners and go over the aspects of our conditioning and experiences.

The reasons why you are overweight are very alike in most people. It is a combination of specific factors coming together. Some persons have more of one type of challenge than another, but the basics are the same.

Many of our weight loss specialists use our mind training audio's additionally to their work because it gives them the added security of knowing that many more aspects are covered than they could in a few one on one sessions.

Step 1 is completed! You are reading this book

The Universe has conspired to get this book into your hands. You can now make the next steps and start accessing the resources hidden in you and learn How to be Slim forever. If you are willing to take the next step, commit and act—your success is guaranteed.

I want to start losing weight now!

We know that most of you will not read the entire book. Statistics show that readers only rarely get beyond the first few chapters of any book. So we won't take it personally if you decide not to read the complete book. In our busy world with an overflow of information, it can be hard to keep our focus and it's all too easy to get sidetracked.

So if you are keen to get started right away and want to get the most out of this revolutionary "Sleep Your Fat Away!" approach to weight loss, go to our website: WWW.SleepYourFatAway.com; get the complete package and embark on your journey towards a healthy, slim body today. Our package contains everything you need to

- Erase the faulty programming of your mind, which is keeping you stuck in bad eating habits and struggling with weight loss
- Train your brain and subconscious mind to support your weight loss and maintain your ideal weight for life
- Align you with your body's intelligence and listen to your body's needs
- Make healthy eating choices
- Enjoy moving more
- Sleep better and wake up feeling refreshed and energized
- And you will receive tips from us and the latest news and updates!

Manipulation is the rule

Our body takes years of consuming more than you need to make it seriously overweight, it does not happen overnight. By being consistent in our bad habits we succeed in creating more weight than is good for us. We eat foods that are processed and refined, in quantities that lead to insulin resistance.

Insulin resistance is when the body cannot handle the sugars any more and the extra is turned into fat. This is one of the major reasons for becoming overweight.

The food industry manipulates the molecules to create a so-called "bliss point." This gives the brain an impulse that will make us crave more of that food (normally these are foods only have minimal amounts of useful nutrients). With clever advertisements they hypnotize us to buy worthless, chemically manipulated foods to excite our palate and brains.

Laziness

We have lost our naturally inborn desire to move our bodies in ways that are consistent with our genetic make-up (deep down we are still hunter-gatherers!). The older we get, the lazier we become. We are glued to our chairs staring at computer screens in a hunched position that causes our discs to degenerate and our backs to become stiff and rigid. With coffee, snacks and sugared drinks readily at our disposal we literally nurture ourselves into bigger masses of biological matter.

Food to manipulate our feelings

To make matters worse we cleverly suppress our emotions with carbohydrates and other foods or drinks. We become numb to the stress caused by our limited ability to behave in an emotionally adult way and take over responsibility for our feelings.

False beliefs

Because of the misinformation given to us by the media and the food and diet industry we believe that losing weight is just a matter of restricting calories, or eating low fat or diet-products. To make matters worse, celebrities get paid very well to become the spokesperson for a diet-brand and as a result many people will continue with the law of insanity: "Doing the same thing over again and expect a different result".

Mind over matter

In this book we will uncover many parts of the puzzle, but most importantly you will get the tools to be able to influence your body's metabolism and cravings better. You can melt your fat away while you sleep!

One of the inborn systems we have not learned to use properly is: our mind. The mind acts like a filter, which limits us in accessing our resources instead of inspiring us to reach for our true potential. This is because by the time we have learned to communicate fluently, we have been conditioned so deeply by our environment: Our families, peers and friends telling us many millions of times who we are, what we can do and mostly: what we cannot do. This makes us develop mainly false and limiting beliefs and these block us from using our mind in an appropriate way and be in control of our bodies.

Step 2: Claim your control and power back!

The goal of this book and the programs we have created is to give you back the control of your body and expand its lifespan and vitality way beyond the normal statistics.

So if you want to be slim, healthy, and vital and have the determination to condition your mind and body: this is the right book for you. Not only will you lose weight, you will also be able to change other areas of your life and achieve more of your goals.

Step 3: Buy a journal and assess where you are now

Make it your personal weight loss journal! Start by answering the questions in the addendum to find out more about your present state before you begin with reading this book.

Warning

1. This book is not a fairy tale nor is it magic. It is based on scientific principles and decades of studying the brain and how to use the power of your mind to change your unconscious habits.

2. This book is not a sales pitch for a special miracle pill or a new fad of weight loss world.

3. This book is related to a product, which you can buy separately. In this book we will explain all the background info and principles you need to understand to execute this new approach. If you go to our website you will get a few free products to get started and test the program. This is where you can get slim now: www.sleepyourfataway.com

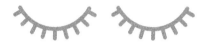

1

Why Depriving Yourself Makes You Fat:
Discover the Difference Between Emotional Hunger and Real Hunger

As babies we naturally follow our inborn survival system. When we are hungry, we cry to let our mums know our stomach is empty and hopefully our mums feed us. Once we have had enough, we stop drinking. Period.

If you have ever tried to feed a new born baby more than it is hungry for, you will know: A healthy baby will refuse to drink if it is not hungry and if it is force fed, it will most likely vomit. The body still naturally eliminates what is too much.

Unfortunately most parents are not educated to really tune into their babies' needs, and so we have the tendency to overfeed our children early on. It's a combination between the idea of showing love via the vehicle of food, the fear of not giving our children enough and also because it's usually the fastest and easiest way to stop a child crying: put some food in their mouth! Adding to that babies can be hard to read and if you have a high maintenance baby, are stressed out by not sleeping enough yourself, you will do anything to get some extra hours of peacefulness… and using food as a handy way of comfort is often the preferred choice of action. Even if a cuddle or some extra attention would have done the trick.

Johnnie's story

Johnnie was a friend I had in elementary school. He was overweight from the day we first met and I saw him growing over the years. I often visited him as he lived just next door and we played together often. He had 3 brothers. All kids were overweight and so were father and mother. At that time I was living on Aruba, also known as the "happy island." At our home we were conditioned to have 3 meals a day, in the morning it was oatmeal (and we ate lots of that!), lunch was normally bread that we took to school in a lunch box and in the evening it was animal protein, with rice, or potato and some salad. In between we never had snacks or anything else to eat. The reason I loved to go play with Johnnie was that they had "eat when you want policy" and there were always snacks available: potato chips, candy, cookies, etc. Besides that, their Mom was always to be found in the kitchen where she was cooking up something to eat. She loved to call us inside to taste her home made snacks, which could be fried fish, fried polenta, fried banana chips, French fries. Each afternoon there was what she called a warm snack. The weekends were terrific as there will be several 'fresh snacks' coming. Her rule was; you should never be hungry and because we played a lot of physical games, we "needed" good food so we would not get skinny. They were of native Indian descendants (Arowaks), who tend not to be so tall and like many South Americans can have the tendency to become quite obese. I was in intense sports, playing tennis almost every afternoon for 2-3 hours straight or attending martial arts classes. The boys next door would play on the street: soccer, basketball with lots of resting periods. Johnnie's mother solved everything with food. This was how she was brought up and that was tradition. If you felt bad you ate; if you felt good you ate; if you lost a game you ate; if you won a game you ate; all the roads led to eating: no exceptions. His baby brother was always walking around in diapers and a bottle of milk; his bottle would be refilled once it was done to 1/3. The baby's name was Camino; he was overweight before he could walk. I am 60 years old. Sadly, Johnnie died at 52 years of a heart attack. At his funeral there was so much finger licking food that even I over indulged in the memory of Johnnie. I was amazed to see how the family I had not seen in a decade hadn't changed one bit, except for being even more overweight! They are a good example of how these habits can completely take over your system and for lots of people it seems like there is no way out. They have lost contact with their body's innate intelligence!

Reconnect with your Body's Intelligence

Because we were often overriding our body's messages for years, it can take a time for us to learn to listen again. It's all about tuning into the real needs of our body and mind; being able to tell the difference between an emotional need such as appreciation, comfort, love and a physical need such as hunger, thirst or movement.

At the beginning it can be hard to differentiate between hunger coming from your stomach ("real" hunger) and your head just *thinking* it is hungry. With head hunger your body is not the one demanding energy…usually something else has triggered you into thinking that food is the answer. This can for example be pure habit ("But *I always eat at little something at 10 o'clock…. or I need to snack whilst watching television…*"), boredom, or stress. Emotional hunger comes rapidly – as opposed to real hunger, which develops slowly. It is important that you learn to tell the difference between these types. Emotional hunger is wired in your brain and when it is triggered by an event or simply because it is time, a cascade of chemical reactions in your brain get you to eat or snack. Sometimes it is simply that you are thirsty and need water, sometimes it is because your blood sugar is low and you need to move your body to get the circulation up so the sugar is released out of the muscles and liver (where it is stored as glycogen). Emotional hunger is a mechanism wired in your brain to eat when you feel emotional or bored and you can change that mechanism!

If you have detected real hunger: EAT! We don't want you to override this need but we do want you to eat consciously, without any distraction and stop when you are full.

The 3 D trigger words: red flags for your mind!

We like comparing our subconscious mind to a gigantic, child like processor. Our subconscious mind records every sound, smell, taste, feeling, and experience we ever had. It not only stores this enormous amount of data but also makes often totally irrational connections between certain words, memories, and actions.

For example: If you as a child once ate a food that was rotten/bad and got sick from eating it, you are very likely to create an aversion to that food and might even stick to it for life.

Or if you had a painful experience, which was linked to a certain smell, you will get an uncomfortable feeling as soon as you smell that smell again – even if it is years later. It can also be a story you have heard, for example it is known that chocolate factories are infested with cockroaches and that the companies are allowed to have up to 0.4% of roaches in their chocolate. For many people their disgust for cockroaches is greater than their desire for chocolate and knowing that fact turns them off! So next time you have that crunchy feeling when eating chocolate you may wonder what it was that you just bit on.

The same applies for certain words! We have discovered 3 strong trigger words connected to the topic of weight loss:

- Diet
- Deprivation
- Discipline

These 3 words can make your subconscious mind throw a fit, tantrum and sabotage your weight loss goals. We tested the effect of these words on hundreds of our clients and discovered that every single one of them reacted strongly to at least two of them. What does this mean for you? As soon as your subconscious mind hears one of the above words or is led to believe something will lead to the 3 D's, it will almost automatically create resistance and start the sabotage process within you. As much as you consciously may want to go on a diet, are ok with depriving yourself of certain foods and being disciplined—your subconscious mind does NOT want to do this. Try it out: Take a few deep breaths in and out; calm your mind and close your eyes. Go into that neutral space inside of yourself and notice how you feel. Become aware of your body and breath and make sure you feel peaceful or at least neutral. Now think of the words: diet, deprivation, and discipline. How do these words make you feel? Are you excited, happy and can't wait to get started? Or do they make you feel slightly reluctant, stressed or even depressed? More than likely it will be closer to the second category.

This is why in Sleep Your Fat Away we don't want you to start out with depriving yourself. We want you to first learn to listen to your body and reconnect to its wisdom. Although we have included some general advice on food (such as to chose natural, organic food whenever possible and stay away from sugar) we want you to eat what you like. As you continue with our program and training your brain, you will automatically eat less and chose for more healthy foods.

Joy's sugary story

When I started to pay attention to my snacking habits I found out that I would crave sugary foods like chocolate whenever I felt overwhelmed. Every time I would go through some stressful periods where my workload was getting more than I could mentally handle, my desire to devour Peanut Butter Cups or Chocolate Mints would soar. My mind had made a strong connection between the feeling of comfort and chocolate. When I grew up my parent's were keen on providing a healthy diet. So there were no sweets to be had in our home and we were also not allowed to eat in between meals. I remember my mum saying: "If you're hungry, you'll eat a piece of dry bread." I also keenly remember how unattractive that dry bread option was to me and how much I would have preferred to have 6 little meals rather than the 3 big ones we were served. I had to force myself to eat breakfast and found it hard to wait for the evening meal, feeling half starved in the late afternoon. So my "solution" was similar to Roy's: I was also lucky to have friendly neighbors, whose mum would serve unlimited breads with butter and sugar sprinkled on top. Now that was yummy!

When we spent all our vacations at our grandparent's house it was like being in paradise. They had the famous "sweety-drawer", filled with delicious chocolate and candy, to which we had unlimited access. Now guess who put on several pounds every vacation and turned into quite a round 10-14 year old?

You see, as soon as my natural young child's desire to move and play active games/sports went down and I replaced it with more "big girl" activities like reading, hanging out, i.e. not moving and still ate more sugary snacks than were good for me. Only when I hit puberty and became more interested in my looks, did I change my eating habits. But it took me all my willpower to get slim and I was still very, very fond of my chocolate. In all honesty, I would prefer to eat a bar of chocolate to having a cooked meal if any one would let me.

Sugar causes all kind of havoc in our brains and its effects on our brain are often compared to those of cocaine. There is a lot scientific data proving that the tremendous intake of sugar is the real cause of our society becoming fatter and sicker every year. I urge you to look into this subject and make the test.

After I learnt all about the sugary evil I decided to confront this demon. Although I was not overweight, I noticed how my energy levels would drop after meals high in carbohydrates. Sometimes I felt like going straight to sleep after a meal. Additionally I noticed how my mood swings were connected to my chocolate consumption. As delicious as the chocolaty treat would taste, it would only offer me a short high and then I would dip into a tired, crabby coma-like state. I tried to eat less sugar frequently and would sometimes succeed to do so for a few days but as soon as the old trigger of overwhelm appeared, so would my "need" for a sugary fix.

Eventually I had had enough of this vicious cycle and decided to put our Sleep Your Fat Away principles to the test on myself. I asked Roy to do a special brain training session on me, where we instilled an aversion to sugar in my mind. After that I listened to this audio and the generic Sleep Your Fat Away sleep program for 10 days. During this time I decided to go off sugar completely. I tossed every single chocolaty and sweet temptation from our home—much to my children's dismay—and replaced them with natural foods such as fruit. And I was amazed at how easily we all adapted. We found it much easier to eat NO sugar than to eat a little sugar. My experience stunned me: I had way more energy, left meals feeling light and ready to go instead of tired and matt. My mood was stable, PMS vanished, and I generally felt more in control.

I stuck to my strict no-sugar-diet for over a month and cannot remember feeling that good in a long time. When I finally had my first ice cream I was astounded to discover that I couldn't finish it. The first few bites tasted good but I quickly had enough and threw the rest away. Now that had never happened to me before! Ever since my sugar fast I have found my taste buds and general way around sugar have changed dramatically. I do indulge in dessert and sugar every once in a while but not nearly as often as I used to and definitely in much, much smaller amounts.

My tip to you:

Once you feel confident with the guidelines and structure our program and have established some new, healthy eating habits, quit sugar for 10 days. Join forces with your friends and/or colleagues and start a no-sugar-challenge. Use the tools we give you in our Sleep Your Fat Away program to balance your emotions and train your brain. Because we know how life changing this choice can be, we have created a special audio to specifically help you combat your sugar addiction. This way you will find it easy to kick the sugar habit!

The 3 D's trigger reactions

The word diet triggers us because it contains a combination of all 3 D's: Diet, Deprivation, and Discipline. We will deprive ourselves for a certain length of time of the foods and snacks we crave and like, and that requires willpower (discipline). Some will also combine this with more exercise to speed up weight loss. Discipline is connected to a time when had to learn the rules and follow them; all the things we liked were not allowed, like watching TV till late at night, eating what we want and when we want; staying in bed; not going to school etc. We had to brush our teeth, take showers and many more things that were not always convenient for us. So discipline led to deprivation of our basic needs and we have stored this link to our memories. So any time the subconscious mind becomes aware of the 3 D's it remembers the time we were not in control and dependent on the good will of our parents and other caretakers. So sabotage starts immediately when our mind thinks we are back in our child years, where we had no control. Our mind will immediately go into resistance mode and fight that choice—no matter how good it is for us. That is why the brain needs to be re-trained in working with you instead of against you!

Simple steps for combating emotional hunger:

✓ Drink a glass of warm water—slowly

✓ Tap your Emotional Balance "stress" point (above your lips, under your nose, in that dent in the middle). See the video on our website

✓ Focus on taking some deep, conscious breaths

✓ Sense which emotion has triggered the feeling of hunger

✓ Accept that feeling and do the Emotional Balance Havening Technique. See the video on our website.

✓ Change focus, distract yourself

✓ Exercise: take a walk, stretch…

✓ Tell yourself it will pass and decide to wait another 10 minutes before reacting

✓ If after doing all the above and having waited for 10 minutes you still feel the need for some food: eat a small portion of something nutritious, such as a handful of almonds, a whole wheat cracker or an apple.

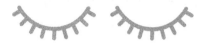

2

It's Not <u>What</u> You Eat but <u>How</u> You Eat:
Utilizing the Secret of Tibetan Monks and Yogis

Think of what yogis and Tibetan monks look like… we have never seen an overweight one. They are all slim, look happy, and usually live very long lives.

What is their secret? It is simple! They treat their food with respect; they take time to say a prayer and to feel gratitude <u>before</u> they take their first bite. Most importantly: they take their time to enjoy their food, they never eat in a hurry, they allow their taste buds to experience the aromas, spices and chew each bite until it is turned into pure liquid. You'll never see them eat in a 'by the way' manner, while doing something else. When they eat, they eat. Period. Also, they never overeat but stop when they feel they have had enough. In this chapter we will train you in these simple strategies to lose weight and keep it off. At the end of this chapter you are on your way to become a naturally slim person for the rest of your life… just by following these guidelines! You don't believe us? Follow them for just 10 days and we are certain you will notice a huge difference in the way you eat.

Your guidelines to become a naturally slim person

One of our most important guidelines is: Eat when you are hungry!

What? I am allowed to eat? This part usually confuses all our program participants. Yes, we want you to start listening to the natural intelligence of your body. Part of this is to know when you are *really* hungry. We do not want you to starve yourself but to learn the difference between emotional hunger and real hunger. Make the test and think of the 3 D's: Diet, Deprivation, and Discipline. How do these 3 words make you feel? Hardly exhilarated, right? The reason is that your mind immediately creates the initiation of a sabotage protocol. We will delve into this mechanism later!

In order to make this program even more effortless and create a lasting change in your lifestyle and eating habits, we are introducing a set of very simple rules to keep to that do not trigger the 3 D's. To support you also on a subconscious level, we have also put these in the audios. This way you are programming your mind to replace the old conditioning and what you think you know about weight loss with more useful and empowering information. These rules are very powerful and easy to remember!

With these 5 guidelines you would be able to lose weight even if you were not to train your brain and do the sleep programming. So if you do not have the money or do not want to invest in yourself, these guidelines will help you to develop the habits of most naturally slim people.

There are 4 types of naturally slim people

- Those who naturally listen to their bodies and without knowing they follow most of these guidelines we will share with you.
- Those that have an extremely high metabolism (you see this in teenagers). They will totally disregard these guidelines and still remain thin. But you may rightly ask yourself if they are *healthy* skinnies. Especially teenagers go through phases of eating masses of junk food.

(Our 4 boys would delight in showing us the thrills of a high sugar, high junk diet if we were to let them!)

- People with a disorder such as a hyper-thyroidism and other medical problems. Some people also seem to have it genetically programmed in them to stay thin no matter what they eat. Some even have problems putting on weight!
- Some people react with stress by not eating or eating less.
- Extreme sports fanatics and bodybuilders. Most aerobic instructors are thin, marathon runners are thin; they burn so many calories that they stay slim.

Copy these guidelines out on sticky notes and stick on your desk, mirror etc. to remind yourself of them at all times! You can also put them on the back of your business card and carry them with you in your wallet. This way you see them often and they become a part of your new, healthy life style.

Guideline #1:

WHEN YOU ARE HUNGRY: EAT!

This is not a diet—you get to eat when you are hungry! No starving, no depriving yourself. Starving yourself is not an option for many reasons.

One is that people who go on a drastic low calorie diet are even more prone to the yo-yo effect and usually put on more weight after ending the diet.

Which is why you don't want to starve yourself but rather reprogram yourself and your eating habits in a healthy way. You want to reset your body and mind to its naturally functional mode. In order to do so you must listen to your body's messages.

When your stomach is empty and needs refueling, you give it what it wants and you EAT! You can eat whatever you want as long as you eat slowly and consciously. Also drink a glass of water before you start to eat.

But: EAT ONLY WHEN YOU ARE REALLY HUNGRY!

Eat when you feel **real** hunger, if you feel emotional; balance yourself and your emotions with the techniques we teach you first. Try not to eat in between your main meals to avoid snacking. Make sure that you eat until you feel comfortable. You can eat whatever you want. If you get hungry for emotional reasons or because you are bored use the Emotional Balance immediately until the emotional hunger goes to zero.

Guideline #2:

EAT WHAT YOU LIKE

This is not a diet, in the sleep programming you will gradually get a craving for natural healthy foods, so in the beginning don't worry about the food you eat, just avoid sugar, snack and chocolate as meals. This rule only works if you eat slow, if you eat fast this rule cannot work and you will not feel what the bad foods do to you. By eating slowly and consciously you will be able to enjoy the food and you will start disliking unhealthy foods. Try to eat French fries slowly; the taste of the grease is not pleasant. Gradually your taste for food will change. Don't count calories, is totally unnecessary, no naturally thin person counts calories.

Guideline #3:

SLOW DOWN!

EAT SLOWLY AND CONSCIOUSLY

Quit eating while doing other things! No more eating in front of the television, reading the newspaper, or checking your mails.

If you are shoveling in food whilst doing something else your brain finds it hard to notice when you are full – it is as if you are eating under trance. It is the same when you watch TV, let's say a football match and you are completely hypnotized by it and whilst watching you are eating popcorn, before you know it the bucket will be empty but you will not notice that it fulfilled you. Distractions help us to eat more because we lose contact with our bodies. This takes the most discipline but is the foundation for success! If you succeed in eating slow you will win the weight loss game with or without sleep programming.

The quickest way to minimizing the amount of food you are eating is by maximizing the time you spend eating it.

Enjoy every mouthful of food, slow down your eating – take those extra minutes, don't rush and chew your food properly (15 times a mouthful).

Put your fork/spoon/knife/sandwich down while you are chewing your food! The reason for this is that it takes a while for the body to send the hormones from your stomach to your brains, telling you that your stomach is full. In the time that it takes for this message to arrive and for you to feel it, you could have eaten much more than is good for you. This is more the norm than an exception. That is why slow eaters are, in general, thinner than fast eaters.

Guideline #4

STOP EATING AS SOON AS YOU FEEL COMFORTABLE

The best way of control is to leave food on your plate. You have to learn that you are the boss over your body and that you are in control. Leaving food on your plate is transcending your past conditioning and breaking free from the years of being told what to do. You will find this easy to do if you eat slowly. You are retraining your mind and body to realize when you are full. Your stomach needs time to register that FULL feeling and send the message to your brain. Whilst in the past your stomach sent your brain the FULL signal, you learn or were taught to override it. Also when you eat too fast, due to the time delay, you will have been continuing to eat although your stomach has had enough. Now it is time to allow your brain and stomach to communicate, to become conscious of the FULL signal, and stop immediately when you get it.

Guideline #5

DRINK LOTS OF WATER!

Water is your best friend; it will reduce your hunger and increase the metabolic rate so you can burn fat more effectively. Water helps to flush your toxins out of your body. In the morning you drink warm water with a lemon to stimulate your digestion, but you will also benefit from a whole list of other vitalizing bonuses. It's as simple as boiling a pot of water, and adding a slice of lemon! Also we tend to mistake thirst for hunger and when you drink a lot you will be less hungry!

Bonus Guidelines

LISTEN TO THE AUDIOS

The audios utilize a wide range of the latest mind management techniques and are an essential part of our work together. It is crucial that you listen to the daytime audios at least once a day (the more often, the better!) and the sleep program for a minimum of 28 days up to 100 days. By listening to the audios your brain is creating new neural pathways in relation to your eating habits and your attitude towards food.

BUY SOMETHING NEW

The law of concentrated attention is one of the most powerful techniques we will be using during this program. It basically boils down to:

If there is something you really want to achieve or have in life then behave as if you already have it.

Your job now is to go out and purchase a new item of clothing in the size that you want to be. It has to be something really new and not something that you have "outgrown." This item of clothing is your goal and I want you to hang it on the outside of your closet/wardrobe – somewhere you can see it often. This visual anchor will help you stay on track. Every time you look at it, take a moment to dwell in some positive feelings, images of how wonderful you will feel and look wearing that piece of clothing.

Note: Interestingly enough our surveys show that people who didn't do this did not lose as much weight as those who did. So don't skip this part!

Here some tips from other experts.

6 Ways to Tap Into Your Hunger Cues

Is your stomach growling or are you being tempted by the sight or smell of food? Here's how to tell and a few tricks to prevent overeating.

We don't always eat because we're hungry. We eat for a number of different reasons, including external cues such as the sight or smell of food. "It's been suggested that we make somewhere close to 200 eating decisions a day," says Edward Abramson, PhD, a clinical psychologist in San Francisco and author of the new book, *It's NOT Just Baby Fat: 10 Steps to Help Your Child to a Healthy Weight*, "and physical hunger is a minority of them."

It's no surprise: We're bombarded by food commercials and ads on billboards and in newspapers and magazines. And because we have such easy access to food with grocery stores and restaurants open 24/7, we can think we're hungry even though we're not, hampering weight loss. "Images in commercials can sensitize the brain as effectively as having the food in front of you," explains Stella Metsovas, CCN, a nutritionist in private practice in Laguna Beach, California.

We also eat in response to emotional turmoil. "We eat to make ourselves feel better when we're anxious or depressed," Abramson says. Emotional eating is more common among women than men, but men do it too, he adds.

How to Stop Eating When You're Not Really Hungry

Studies have shown that if we listen to our body's signals about hunger, fullness, and appetite, we will know better when to stop eating. And weight loss is easier when you listen to what your body is telling you. This is the reason why the virtual gastric band is so effective; it is the easiest way to get back in touch with your body's intelligence.

These tips can help you get back in touch with your body and know when you're truly hungry, so you will eat at the right times and boost your efforts to lose weight:

Keep a journal. Write down how you feel after consuming a large meal. "It will help you to correlate any food hangovers with overeating," Metsovas says. It's easy to keep a food log. "It doesn't have to be too elaborate — maybe a 3" by 5" card that has the time of day and where and what you were eating and how you felt," Abramson suggests. "After a week, look at it and see if there are any obvious patterns." If you notice that you're overeating or eating unhealthy foods when you sit down to watch TV at night, you may be able to switch to healthier fare, such as air-popped popcorn rather than a buttered version, or find something else to do with your hands, such as knitting or crocheting.

Don't sit down for a meal starving. You can help curb your appetite by drinking water or sipping herbal tea before a meal. If you're truly hungry and dinner isn't for another hour or so, have a small snack, such as a handful of almonds or pretzels or cut-up veggies with low-fat dressing.

Eat frequent small meals. "It's often helpful for anyone trying to lose weight to go on interval eating — have a mini-meal every 3 to 3½ hours throughout the day," says Daniel C. Stettner, PhD, director of psychology at UnaSource Health Center in Troy, Mich., and an adjunct professor at Wayne State University in Detroit. The key is to keep meals *mini* if you're going to eat more frequently. Otherwise, you'll be overeating.

Take 20. "A meal ideally needs to be 20 minutes or longer," Stettner says. "Twenty minutes is the magic number because it takes 20 minutes for the stomach to send signals to the brain to let it know you are eating. If you scarf food down in 5 to 10 minutes, your brain hasn't caught up yet with your stomach. If you stretch a meal to 20 minutes or longer, it makes it more satisfying and you feel fuller."

Play detective. Ask yourself these questions: "Why am I eating this? Am I truly hungry? Do I feel light-headed because I haven't eaten for a while? Or am I eating because the clock says it's time? Am I craving something sweet because I'm upset about a problem?" Knowing why you're eating gives you the opportunity to make an informed decision about whether you want to eat versus automatically eating something, Abramson says.

Be discerning about dessert. Studies have shown that if you eat chocolate when you're hungry, you have less control, so you'll eat it faster and consume more." If you really like chocolate chip cookies, save them for dessert," Abramson says. "If you eat your treats at the end of a meal as dessert, it decreases the strength of future cravings for them. I can't tell you the mechanism of why this is so, but studies show it's a way of reduced cravings."

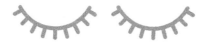

3

Regain Control of your Life by Unleashing the Power of your Mind

Therapy versus Coaching

There is a big difference between coaching and therapy. Coaching is taking someone who is coach-able, committed and motivated to make the necessary changes in their life, through a series of interventions by a trained professional, to where they can access more of their potential (resources). Coaching has become a highly paid profession in top sports as it became clear that athletes perform much better when supported by coaches. Then it went on to the area of coaching executives in businesses and started trickling down to the more motivated people in the community. Nowadays many people have coaches and because of that they perform better, achieve more of their goals and overcome their challenges more easily. Joy and Roy only coach people who are seriously committed to clear goals. We work with CEO's, top-athletes, celebrities, and other achievers. Therapy is normally the way to go when there is a mental, emotional, or physical problem that you cannot solve yourself and you seek outside professional help. This can be a psychotherapist, medical professional or even a naturopathic physician or healer.

Here a quick overview of the differences:

COACHING VS. THERAPY

- Creating the future vs. Healing the past
- Building momentum vs. Trying to get comfortable
- Commitment to a specific measurable result vs. Wanting relief
- Generating tangible results vs. Attempting to get rid of unwanted things
- Being bold and ready now vs. Making only the necessary changes to get well
- Speaking about desired outcomes vs. Talking about things in order to feel better
- Thriving vs. Surviving
- Playing big and bold vs. Taking careful, small steps
- Being assertive and proactive vs. Trying to handle past consequences
- Focus on creating value vs. Focus on being helped or "saved"
- High intention behaviors vs. High drama behaviors
- Living out of powerful declarations vs. Living out of dis-empowering stories
- Acting powerfully in spite of unwanted thoughts, feelings & emotions vs. Working to get rid of unwanted thoughts, feelings & emotions
- Achieving goals vs. Getting fixed

What you see is that therapy is often a reaction to something you don't want (you want to let go of) whereas coaching is to move to a higher level of manifestation or your potential. When I (Roy) saw that most therapies keep the patient dependent and often in a victim role, I created a new approach we called Omega Health Coaching. Here we use the principles of coaching and apply them to people with disease.

Our aim is to give them:

1. Control over their life (as a part of the healing)
2. The tools and techniques to become self-responsible and self-healing
3. o keep them accountable for their actions and input instead of them entirely depending on what the therapist is doing

Every patient/client got homework, things to do; to assist in the healing process and train their minds and brains for success. We coached them to be focused on <u>what they want</u> rather than on <u>what they don't want</u>! This was a big revolution in Europe and radically changed the way of natural healing. Some of the most powerful tools we found to give the control back to the client were hypnosis and self-hypnosis (listening to audio-recordings that teach you to take back control of your mind and body).

Elisabeth's story

Elisabeth is a beautiful blonde Italian accountant (in her 40's) and a frequent visitor of our workshops on healing and personal development. She once said to me: "What really changed my life was when I understood that any disease is a chance to look at what you need to change in your life and what you really want out of life. Before I came to your workshops I was living on autopilot. I had a good business and a lot of nice things but on the other side I had a lousy relationship with lots of tension. But I thought that it was normal to be stressed by work and your relationship; all my friends were in the same boat! But then one day I started getting headaches, then insomnia and finally pain in my neck. My life became miserable. I was taking loads of pills, got a stomach ulcer, and was very tired. Work became an effort and my business was going down, as I could not put in the hours I did before. Then a friend of mine came back from a weekend with you and she was dramatically changed, started to meditate and listen to your audios. She went from being depressed and overweight to being happy, slim, and dynamic in just 3 months time! She even lent me some of her Omega Healing CD's and I was delighted. After 2 weeks I was sleeping better, I got off the pills I was taking and decided to come to your and Joy's workshops. That was 2 years ago. My whole life has changed!

I am now divorced and happy. My ex-husband and I are at peace with each other. My business is booming and my child is far happier as there is no more tension at home. In the weekends he is with his father, who is now also coming to your workshops since he saw what happened with me. We are all better off, thank you, thank you!"

The most important tool that made the big transformation in Elisabeth's life was claiming her power back and realizing that she had the capability to create the life she wanted. She achieved this mainly with the (self) hypnosis techniques we use.

Why Using Hypnosis is like Unleashing Rocket Power Within You! What is Hypnosis?

<u>Hypnosis</u> happens any time we are relaxed and (consciously or subconsciously) open our minds. In this state we bypass our critical thinking to receive information that we accept at a deeper level. When we are in a relaxed state we can access what is in our subconscious mind! Some people are much more suggestible than others. Everyone is suggestible and can be influenced with positive or negative information. The most important thing is that the new information does not conflict with strong convictions such as our moral values as this will make us reject it. If it contradicts our morals or religious beliefs we can immediately shut down and reject the information even when we are confronted with solid evidence. The brain will come up with a rationalization why it cannot work. So for us to accept the information it needs to work with our strongest beliefs and morals. That is the reason why you cannot have someone do something against his or her convictions. For example, if you hypnotize a soldier and tell them that they have to kill someone because he is an enemy, the soldier will probably do that. If you do the same with a person who is against killing, you cannot get them to kill another person!

<u>Conversational hypnosis</u> happens when you trust and respect someone or you consider them to be an authority than you are much more likely to accept their suggestions. As a parent we give many suggestions to our children, also reinforce the behavior we like and punish the behavior we don't want. This way we influence them and instill beliefs, behaviors, and habits in them.

Our tone of voice and the speed with which we talk can have a hypnotic effect! Also when we are confused and have to think about something we are unconsciously more open to receive new information.

Our teachers are trusted authorities and can have tremendous hypnotic effects on the mind of their students. Other sources of hypnosis are people we look up to: doctors, celebrities, icons, teachers, etc.

The power of media and TV is well documented; they are the most damaging hypnotic sources known to mankind.

Doctors can hypnotize a person without them realizing and thus influence their realities. If a doctor tells you that you have an incurable condition and that it will get worse over time, this will increase the probability of that happening! There are reports of people dying because they got the wrong diagnosis and heard they will die within a certain period of time. Because they accepted that suggestion to be true, they subconsciously created that reality and fulfilled their own prophecy.

A similar effect has been documented in some primitive cultures where a shaman cursed a person to die (just with words!) and the person than would fall down dead just because they believed the shaman had powers over them! Words can be very powerful and influence you more than you realize.

Therapeutic hypnosis: the main use of hypnosis is to support someone to undo the barrage of negative suggestions they received in their lifetime, especially in their younger years when they were against all the information coming in. Over time these suggestions have formed their self-image. Hypnosis is the fastest way to do that because it brings them back to the same receptive state they were in when they received and accepted the negative information. The hypnotist builds up a level of trust with the client, assists them to get in a relaxed state and bring them in a 'sleep' like state where they are more receptive. Hypnosis has an effect on the brainwaves: the client goes from an awakened brain state (also called beta brainwaves) to a relaxed state (alpha brainwaves) to a deeply relaxed state (theta brainwaves). The same pattern is seen when we go to sleep. The difference is that when we sleep, we lose contact with the external world and go inside of our minds without any external input. Sounds outside of us (that are not familiar) may startle us awake. In hypnosis, the hypnotist maintains contact with the client so they do not fall asleep but keep following the voice of the hypnotist. During hypnosis you usually have short bursts where you drift away, then you hear the voice again and you follow the voice of the hypnotist. Because you are relaxed and trust the hypnotist, you are open to change and that is why you can accept the suggestions given to you by the hypnotist.

Another great advantage of hypnosis is that we have access to our memories and we can be guided to go back to certain events that happened in our lives. We can, under guidance of the hypnotist, change the meaning we give to these events. This is one of the most powerful healing effects of hypnosis. You can change limiting beliefs into empowering beliefs.

Using hypnotic suggestions without a hypnotist

A very powerful hypnotic method that has gained tremendous popularity over the years is listening to special audio recordings. You regularly (normally once a day) listen to positive suggestions that can be very specific to a theme you want to change, for example your self-esteem. On the audio there is usually a first part to relax the person into alpha brainwaves. Then follow positive affirmations in the "I" form or "You" form.

For example: "I am a good person and I love myself"

"I appreciate and value myself"

"I feel good about myself"

Or: "You are a good person and you love yourself"

"You appreciate and value yourself"

" You feel good about yourself"

Another way to reinforce this is to repeat these affirmations in the "I" form on your own as often as possible. If you practice that, it will also have an effect over time, as the subconscious mind start to accept these suggestions to be true and then you start behaving as if they are true.

The positive suggestions need to be repeated over an extended period of time for them to have a lasting effect. It is like a plant that needs to grow roots to become strong and healthy over time. It takes time to create a new self-image and for new behavioral patterns to replace the old ones. The minimum duration time for a full re-conditioning of the subconscious mind is 28 days and it is the bare minimum based on research showing that it takes 28 days to create new habits.

Many hypnotists use audio recording to reinforce their sessions.

After a lot of experimenting we discovered that it is safer to say that it takes on average 90 to 100 days for the suggestions to grow strong roots in the subconscious mind. That is why we prefer 100 days of listening to positive mind programming. It is like growing young trees in a forest, after 28 days they are OK and if nothing bad happens, like a storm or monsoon, you know they will become strong healthy trees. After 100 days however, the roots are so firmly implanted that you know even if a big storm or hurricane comes, the trees will be fine. That is why we go the extra mile and recommend 100 days, even though we know that on average after 28 days all is fine.

Sleep hypnosis and nightly brain training: this is when we listen to positive suggestions during our sleep. During our sleep we have similar brainwave patterns as during hypnosis and we are the most open to receive new information, as we are most relaxed. There are 6 advantages to sleep-hypnosis:

1. The duration is much longer than an average hypnosis session and therefore it is more effective.
2. The client receives many more repetitions than in normal hypnosis or a normal audio session.
3. With our method the client incorporates the suggestions in their dreams and that makes them even more real and creates a better acceptance.
4. It is easy to do, just put the audio on a barely audible volume and go to sleep!
5. You can do it every night and are independent from outside help.
6. It is much cheaper than hypnosis sessions.

Some downsides

There is, however, a caveat: When the audio recording is not specifically developed for sleeping, it can cause people to wake up every hour and they can be come very exhausted from that. Also most people put the volume on too high. It is much better to have it at whisper mode so your subconscious mind picks it up and you bypass the conscious mind much easier. You should barely be able to hear the voice!

Breakthrough

We have pioneered a new way to deliver positive messages during the sleep time to speed up healing, weight loss, positive self-esteem, stop smoking and much more. We call our method "sleep programming"; it includes a special program to create a new approach that we called dream-integration (will be explained in detail later).

Causal hypnosis

Causal hypnosis is when we go back to the exact incident (the cause) that traumatized the person and heal that. Healing happens rapidly when we change the meaning of that incident. This works excellently for phobias and certain emotional patterns. Normally when done correctly, this only needs to happen once. This technique used in hypnosis is called age-regression.

We have applied a special way of age regression, which allows the subconscious mind to go back and change the meaning of the traumatic incidents. This will eventually result in more emotional freedom and happiness.

Spiritual hypnosis

Spiritual hypnosis is based on the concept that we are eternal beings, who incarnate in a body on this planet and have several lifetimes as human beings. It is also to incarnate on other planets. The science of spiritual hypnosis discovered that we have memories of having lived before in previous times. We still carry memories of these lifetimes and some of these memories can be traumatic and influence how we experience certain situations in this lifetime. In this book it is not important to believe about past lives. It is totally irrelevant for the method we have designed. You don't need to believe for this method to work!

The process of bringing a person back to these memories is called regression therapy.

By regressing a person to a time before birth, most people will experience memories that give them the impression they lived before as the images and memories can be very vivid. Traumas and suffering in those lives can leave an imprint that influences the person in their current life negatively. By changing the meaning of the traumas, many persons find that a change takes place in their current lives as well. Many other avenues can be explored such as contact with guides, the Higher Self, in-between-lives memories and more. In our sleep programming this happens automatically by using metaphorical language and allowing the Higher Self to guide the person in their healing process. The subconscious mind speaks another language than the conscious mind and can be directed to do what is necessary to get a certain result. If you tell the subconscious mind to find the very first incident of the traumatic event that is causing the current problem or challenge in their lives, it will go back as far as it can. The subconscious mind is automatically connected with all this information when we are in a deeply relaxed state. This information is not in the body, it is non-local. This means that it is like tuning into a radio station to get certain information. Nowadays we can store our information in an I-cloud or other databases that is not in your computer but can be anywhere on the earth. Through Internet the computer can wirelessly connect to the data storage and recollect that information. Our minds work in a very similar way.

Another form of spiritual hypnosis is taking a person to in-between-lives and allowing them to experience the time before they came into a body.

In the sleep programming we allow the subconscious mind to guide the person to find the causes of weight gain. This is all that is needed for removing the issues that could block losing weight and staying on one's path.

Suggestive hypnosis: The power of suggestion

The power of suggestion is not the privilege of hypnosis; it is part of our daily lives. When people say something bad to you or criticize you, it changes your emotional state. If many people tell you that you look sick, you may find that you feel slightly sick after a few times. If people give you lots of compliments, this elevates your mood and you feel better. Giving compliments and showing appreciation has a very powerful effect on people and can change the way they feel about themselves.

If cancer patients hear a story that someone healed himself or herself from the identical cancer they have by for example eating carrots, they might find healing in eating carrots. And the more people you know with the same stories, the stronger the effect becomes. This is also called the formation of a mass consciousness and belief.

In medicine this power of suggestion is divided in two kinds: the positive effect (placebo) and the negative effect (nocebo)

Placebo: if a client believes or is suggested that some therapy will work, the effects of that therapy is increased even if the therapy itself would have zero effect. Also the suggestions can counteract the chemical effects of medicine. The mind is stronger than the chemical dosage used in medicine. Just wearing a medical looking outfit will increase the effects of a therapy. Placebo is the most scientific proof of the power of hypnosis. The placebo effect has been proven in more than half the medicine to be more powerful than the chemicals itself. (Also see previous chapter)

Nocebo; this is the opposite hypnotic effect of placebo, this is the negative effect caused by the words used by the medical authorities. If the doctor tells the client that they have terminal disease and have only 3 months to live, that has enormous impact on the lifespan of the client and often will shorten their life.

Suggestology: doctors have avoided the use of placebo because they don't believe in it, whilst scientific evidence shows in thousands of research settings that it is the most powerful healing force available to mankind. It is far more powerful than the chemicals doctors prescribe as medicine. (Self) Hypnosis is where the power of the mind is engaged to activate the self-healing and self-regulating mechanisms of the body-mind complex. It is the most effective and fastest way to self-empowerment!

The hypnotic power of surgery: When a client with heart-problems due to narrowed arteries to the heart is operated upon and the skin is cut and closed while they are under anesthesia and they did not receive a bypass (but think they did), the symptoms can disappear as if they received a bypass. The same is the case for painful arthritic knees. In other words if the client believes to be operated upon, it already has a tremendous healing effect.

Implanting an imagined memory: One of the biggest breakthroughs in hypnosis we discovered is that you can make a person believe subconsciously that they had a certain incident happen to them, when in "reality" it did not happen. For example with smokers you can give them the suggestion that they never smoked and erase the memory of them smoking. Technically you are erasing what is called synapses. Synapses are neurological pathways that keep a certain habit on automatic. When that is erased you cannot indulge in that habit automatically anymore. This can be temporary or, with reinforcement, in some cases permanent. You can also create synapses for a new habit and that will with time become automatic.

The possibilities are limitless. You can create an aversion to cigarettes, chocolate, certain foods or the opposite: craving for water, healthy foods, exercise etc.

Weight loss hypnosis: we use a combination of hypnotic techniques and acupressure points to change the behaviors, the emotional causes, the self-image, eating habits and the relationship to food and exercise. One of the highlights of the program is that we implement the memory of a gastric band operation to shrink the stomach. Furthermore the participants have to follow some simple guidelines and practice certain techniques to deal with their emotions. It is not one single hypnosis session but a series of sessions supported by audio-sessions to get long lasting, sustainable, life changing effects. It takes a small commitment from the clients to stick to the program, to change from inside and not to engage in useless calorie restriction diets which would worsen the situation. In 4-5 weeks the foundation is created for a life long continuation of the process and after that it is about reinforcement and maintenance. When done this way the long-term success rate will be above 90%. That is unheard of in the world of weight-loss!

How effective is hypnosis for weight loss?

Clinical research shows around 35% long lasting results with hypnosis. If you privately ask most hypnotists if they see success with weight loss hypnosis, you may be surprised to discover how few actually have long term success with their overweight clients. It is also a very complex process that takes a lot of sessions. That's because they try to change everything but the most basic (and most simple) problem... You cannot program new habits without erasing the synapses that keep the old habits on autopilot! And that is exactly why our program has over 95% success! It is a complete reprogramming package from inside out and does not require will power. The most important part of this program happens during your sleep!

All you need to do is sleep

... And have the brain training (sleep program) running in the background.

Brain Training: Sleep Reprogramming is the answer

To learn new habits, you have to unlearn old habits first. Otherwise you will have to do it with will power and that takes a lot of discipline and most people will not make it. In fact only 4 to 6% succeeds on willpower alone!

With these new techniques your mind will be reprogrammed to its natural, healthy state. Years of negative programming by your parents, teachers, and media will be undone.

For example: "eat all on your plate!" is the most powerful negative anti-natural conditioning that our parents have installed in us. Reprogramming happens when we repeatedly listen to the positive affirmations when we are in a relaxed state (alpha or better theta brainwaves) and not paying attention. We need a minimum of 28 days of unconscious listening in order to create new behaviors, then reinforce that for another 70 days for it to become completely ingrained in the psyche and subconscious mind.

The Virtual Gastric Band

The breakthrough in weight loss was when a British hypnotist (Sheila Granger) started giving suggestions that the client had had a gastric bypass surgery, their stomach was now smaller, and the client could only eat small portions of food! This had immediate effect and people start losing weight effortlessly.

This has been the mayor breakthrough in weight loss and hypnosis. With our techniques you can install a virtual gastric band that will literally shrink your stomach size without any surgery. It will feel as if you have had a real surgical intervention. But it only happened in your imagination. This makes the big difference and with the added strategies you will become a fat-burner instead of a sugar burner. You will be less hungry, feel satisfied faster, plus feel happy and content because your emotional baggage is reduced every day while you listen to the audio-programs.

The secrets of the naturally thin people

We will install in your mind the habits of the naturally thin. The program will delete the habits that have kept you stuck in a cycle of dieting, starving, or binging and create a mental program that will allow you to live like the naturally slim people. So you can eat what you want and still loose weight. So you can stop beating yourself up and start genuinely liking yourself. This combination of a gastric band, reprogramming to your natural state is synergistic and will last you a lifetime.

Eliminate self-sabotage forever

Forget about depriving yourself and learn how to love yourself. We will help you by reprogramming your subconscious mind to be, live, and eat like a naturally thin person. This will result in you stopping with emotional overeating and self-sabotage.

The end result is not only losing weight but also improving the quality of your life in many ways. It is self-empowerment on several levels.

Two ways to go

Work with a hypnotist or coach trained in the How To Be Slim Program (check our website)

Buy our mind reprogramming system and do it at home

Going to the hypnotist

The How To Be Slim expert will normally set up 4 to 5 sessions: The first four within 4 weeks to get the 28-day minimum for changing the subconscious programming. This has the advantage that you can work with your hypnotist on personal issues, especially in the 3rd and 4th sessions. The disadvantage is that there are not many hypnotists that are trained in doing the gastric band method and therefore that option may not be available to you. The costs can be imperative for some people but in the end it is the result that counts.

Light trance: just being relaxed is enough!

Some people are concerned that they will not be able to go into a state of hypnosis. But this is not a big thing in this procedure because it is mainly about you *imagining* going to a hospital and doing the procedure for the gastric band. It does not require a person to go into deep trance; just a little bit of relaxation is enough to get a good effect. The reason for this is that even though the conscious mind knows that in reality the procedure never happened, the subconscious mind believes that it happened and starts to react as if it has happened. You just need to play along. That is all we need to get the results we want. This procedure is effective for 2 reasons:

1. The subconscious mind is more powerful than the conscious mind and has direct influence on our bodily functions.
2. We want it to happen, we don't fight it consciously. We want to change and that makes it even more effective. For these two reasons the gastric band procedure with hypnosis has become one of the most successful techniques in the history of hypnosis.

Programming

Everyone can go in a light trance where the brainwaves are a little bit slower (alpha-state); you don't need to be very good in hypnosis to be able to do that. The hypnotist should make an audio-session for you to listen to every day at home to get the programming effect or they can use one of our recordings. This will enhance the technique and make it even more successful. It is important that the client reinforces the procedure by listening to the audio-sessions every day. This is how you build the synapses in the brain and keep on removing the old conditioning that you have received and keep you imprisoned with habits that no longer serve you and your health.

The sequence

Most hypnotists will do the gastric band in the first session; we prefer the second session to recreate the tension of the real procedure. The 2nd, 3rd and 4th sessions are to work on emotional issues, react to any challenges and to create aversion against unhealthy foods, bad habits and adjust the stomach size if needed. For most people this is all that is needed and the results are phenomenal.

How much weight will you lose?

The amount of weight lost over a certain period varies enormously. Most people from day one are in a rhythm and steadily lose a certain amount per week. Some people start fast and then stabilize to a steady rhythm. Some start slow and speed up later. The main thing to remember is that everyone has his or her own pace. We are in for a steady step by step weight loss that is good for the body to handle and adapt to. That pace is determined by the body's intelligence and is the optimal pace for that person. Gradual weight loss and consistency is better than yo-yoing or plateau-ing!

The end result

One of the questions we were asked:

How is it possible that you can make a product that helps almost everybody? The answer consists of several parts:

1. How much weight do you want to lose?

This is one of the most individual parts and is addressed in our program by having the client focus on the end result. They start each session with stating the end result, and then the subconscious mind is programmed to go for that specific individual result. So the weight loss is exactly programmed for the individual end result. When you reach your desired result you can start with the maintenance program to keep the weight you desire and make sure you don't fall back.

2. Most emotional issues are common

The reasons for over-eating are very common and widespread. A large percentage of people have learned to suppress emotions in ways that are very similar. Boys should not cry, so they learn to suppress their emotions. Girls can cry but get attention when they cry and sometimes are programmed by getting a snack for not feeling good. So they tend to eat when emotional. Than we can develop patterns like eating when bored, depressed, angry, etc. That famous tub of ice cream to alleviate stress in our relationships... The most common emotional patterns are addressed in the weight loss programming and we help the client to change their habitual patterns into healthy ones.

3. The lifestyle of a naturally thin person

A very important part of the program is to re-establish our natural instincts, to only eat when we are hungry and stop eating when we feel satisfied. Little children are born with these instincts. It is through the conditioning of worried parents, ignorant doctors and dieticians that we break the natural patterns and condition patterns that will lead later to weight gain. The gastric band is there to make it easy for the client to return to these natural patterns as they are getting back in touch with their natural instincts.

4. Positive Self image

Another important part of the program is that we have to change the way we see ourselves. Over 80% of the population subconsciously has a negative programming about themselves. That is the reason why most people criticize themselves and often have negative thoughts about themselves and others. The main reason we judge others is because we judge ourselves. Overweight people have a strong tendency to judge and criticize themselves and at the same time that leads to more emotional overeating. It is an important ingredient in the weight loss programming to address this, so that over time our clients start feeling better about themselves. They judge themselves less and this changes their emotional moods and how they feel about themselves.

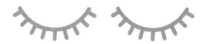

4

Why Being Fat Does Not Have to be Your Karma

What is the karmic story behind being overweight? This chapter is not about spirituality; it's about real, everyday life. The word karma is used for many things.

The word karma is often used in the context of bad karma or good karma, meaning good fortune and bad luck. But in the context of weight loss karma plays another role. So lets start with looking at the meaning of the word "karma."

What is Karma?

Karma is a Sanskrit word and in Indian religions it describes the concept of "action" or "deed," understood as that which causes the entire cycle of cause and effect.

Karma is actually nothing particularly spiritual; it is a scientific principle of cause and effect. If you do A you will get B. On the surface of being overweight it all seems easy and transparent: you can say it is just the consequence of eating more than you need for energy. End of story and that is why the common logical solution is to go on a calorie-restricted diet, take diet pills to numb hunger or block the uptake of fat or carbohydrates and exercise more. But experience shows that these approaches don't work long term for most people.

Why not? That is exactly what this book is about!

Our definition of Karma

Karma is time related (linear effect), but they're a few aspects of karma that may be beyond our normal linear time-line experience.

1. Instant effect

You do something and you immediately get a response. For example you eat something that is not good for you and you become sick and throw up. The direct effect lets you recognize the link between the two events.

2. Delayed effect

You do something and the effect shows up some time later. Here it may be harder to see the correlation between cause and effect. For example a dentist uses anesthesia and you become sensitive to it. So the first time you have no reaction but 2 years later you get the same anesthetic and now you get a strong allergic reaction to it. The same goes for certain foods. You might be able to tolerate them for some time but "suddenly" you become intolerant towards foods you used to enjoy. This can be caused by the general toxicity in your body. Once it reaches a certain level, the body cannot handle it any longer and will react in an allergic way. Many people nowadays become sensitive to gluten and because of that many people feel lethargic and tired but do not know why!

3. Long delayed effect

The effects may show up many years later. For example it takes many years of overeating before you are severely overweight. Or lung cancer can take many decades of smoking before it develops.

4. Non-linear effect

This is a karmic effect we usually don't understand. For example something happens in your family-line (ancestors) and you get the consequences. For example: allergies in your genetic line. So it is not something you did but something you inherit. Some people believe in past life karma. Even though we don't know if that is true and will not go into that, it is something to consider.

Instant karma is never a problem as you get the chance to correct it immediately. The consequences of your action are reflected back to you right away and you can choose what to do next. If everything were instant karma, we would learn fast and it would be easier to stay on our path!

Delayed karma is more difficult to recognize and there may be no recognition of the primary deed causing the effect. It can develop silently over time and sometimes it is even too late when we discover the consequences.

Many of our old age diseases can be explained with the delayed karma-effect and often have nothing to do with old age. One example is bone-demineralization. When you don't exercise, over the years the bones lose calcium and all the sudden at very old age you fall down and, for example, break your hip. This is caused by a lack of exercise and not an old age problem.

Fat is delayed karma made visible

Being overweight is a metaphor for something else, it means that there is something for you to look at and change.

The good thing about being overweight is that it is visible. *You are wearing your karma on your body.* Most other problems are less visible.

Skin cancer and wrinkles can be the karma years of excess sun tanning, some people may be so sensitive that they develop skin cancer without excessive tanning.

Most of the karmic consequences of our life style choices are hidden, for example arterial plaques (the narrowing of the blood vessels that can lead to heart attacks, strokes and other problems). These problems may appear much later in life as memory loss, heart attacks, brain infarctions (stroke) with paralysis on one side, Parkinson's, Alzheimer's, etc.

So if you are overweight the good news is that you can see it and you are aware of having a problem or the beginning of a problem. The bad news is that you have been struggling for some time. You have either given up, or you are still trying things that don't work or believe you do not have the willpower to do it. The other bad news is that you may fall victim of the many weight loss theories and scams that don't work permanently and make you stay stuck in a vicious cycle.

The really good news is that you now have this book and the new system to help you change it.

Fat is secondary karma

Karma is the consequence of our actions or choices, so it seems as if being overweight is just a simple mathematical equation. You consume more calories than your body is processing and that is why the extra amount is stored as energy (fat). That seems simple enough! Most scientists will close the case, leave it at that and say: consume less, burn more calories and the problem is solved. Based on their science the only way to lose the extra ballast is by restricting the caloric intake or by burning more through exercise. This formula works but for most people it is not sustainable long time. There is another problem that keeps throwing them back to consuming more calories than their body needs: when you go for a long time in a state of deprivation (starving) fighting hunger then the body will react by lowering your metabolic rate to conserve energy. The longer they go on a calorie restricted diet, the lower the metabolism. The low metabolism means they are burning fewer calories than they normally would and with less food they will plateau and have difficulties losing weight. The danger is that when you start eating normal again your weight shoots up! Doing the right kind of exercise when you are eating less can prevent this. This way you are also preventing the feeling of deprivation and starvation. All this is included in the guidelines we will give you in this book! So they are stuck in a downward spiral. So what is the other factor that is more primary?

Conditioning #1. Primary Karma for being overweight in this life

All weight problems go back to your conditioning and behavior patterns you learn early on. As a child you were told to eat all of your food even when you felt full, or you were not hungry or did not like the food. You were conditioned to go against your instincts and you learn that you are not right about how you feel in your body. Your parents and/or teachers overruled your self-regulating mechanisms with their power of authority. This is the first big conditioning that occurred and completely deregulated your system. If we don't listen to our bodies, we get trapped in a time related Pavlov-reflex system (you remember that famous dog drooling whenever the bell was rung?). It is lunchtime, you should eat, so you eat, whether you are hungry or not. You go to a restaurant and you get a full plate of food (far more than you need) but you eat it all because you are conditioned to eat everything on your plate. Most people don't eat because they are hungry but because it is time to eat!

Many people eat breakfast even though they are not hungry in the morning. But they were told that breakfast is the most important meal of the day and it was important to eat so you have the energy. That is complete non-sense and there are numerous studies proving this theory wrong. The most important rule is: **Listen to your body**. *If you are not hungry do not eat!* It is totally OK to skip breakfast and even not eat all morning if you feel like it – just make sure you stay well hydrated and drink lots of water. We dive further into this topic in chapter 13.

There are some people who only eat twice a day and are slim, there are also people who eat 6 meals a day and they are slim. What do they have in common? They listen to their bodies, eat when they need it and eat just enough for what their body needs!

A body-builder or athlete who has huge muscles and trains hard may consume 4 times the amount of what a normal person eats and will still not put on weight!

Conditioning #2. The karma of your environment (modern living)

If your parents used a lot of salt or sugar, you will be conditioned to do the same. Certain cultural habits are also added to your conditioning and you will be following in the footsteps of previous generations. But what changed is that you grew up in a different world than your parents did. Maybe your parents had to walk to school and you did not have to. Maybe you played outdoors less than your parents did, maybe they had more siblings than you have, and maybe they had less to eat than you have. There is always a big difference between the generations. For example one generation had less sugar, less meat, less bread. So your conditioning is based on what your parents changed in their habits because the environment changed as well. We now have more sugar than ever, more coffee, more refined foods, more cheese, more margarine, more genetically manipulated foods, more junk food, we eat out more, etc. The agricultural industry depends more on petrochemical fertilizers and pesticides, the cattle get more antibiotics, hormones, and junk food to eat (cows are forced to eat the remainders of other cows). We are exposed to petrochemicals and hormones in our foods that have an endocrinal (hormonal) effect on our bodies and can make us fat.

Also when you move out from your own environment, you can get karma. For example, your children go to study at the University and start eating like other students and party like them. Some people adapt to their partner's habits when they get married. Another classic are the men who gain weight when their wife is pregnant.

One of Roy's sons went to University. He was brought up eating healthy wholesome organic foods, take vitamin pills, drink water, and eat his greens. He was never significantly sick besides having asthma as a child. He went to study for 4 years and went on a student diet of pizzas, refined foods, sweets, soft drinks, and beer, and started smoking. When he came back he was a total mess, stressed, caught colds easily and looked unhealthy. 4 years did more damage than the many years before could to protect him against that environment. It takes time to find your perfect healthy balance and it can be hard.

Conditioning #3. The karma of your learned behavior with foods

If as a child when you cried or were unhappy and your parents or Grandparents gave you sweets to console you, you learn to numb your unhappy feelings with food. Some people discover the power of eating as an antidepressant or as a way to suppress emotions all by themselves. They eat when bored, lonely, sad, frustrated, or angry. This can be another karmic reason for you being overweight. It happens a lot and many people who are overweight suffer from what we call "emotional hunger." This term defines the use of food to deal with emotions or to feel good. Emotional hunger is a prime cause for being overweight. Check chapter 1 again to see how to deal with emotional hunger.

Conditioning #4. The karma of emotional and unresolved traumas

The karmic laws are very simple: you cannot run away from the issues you have to deal with. If you do, you are just pushing the problems into the far future. If you do not deal with the unresolved issues when they surface in your life, they will show up again later for you. Usually in ways that make it virtually impossible to see the connection with the cause. As a rule of thumb: The longer you ignore what you need to learn, the more intense your lessons will become!

For example, if you learn to suppress your anger and you now never get angry, you have become a passive aggressive. This means you express your anger by using sarcasm, judging people, avoiding aggressive people, bad mouthing people behind their backs, etc. You believe you are not an angry person whilst below your calm surface you most certainly are. In our practice we found that around 80% of all cancers have suppression of anger or an unresolved issue as a karmic cause, genetics or toxins can trigger this. The traumas you have not resolved in your youth will always haunt you, no matter where you go. The lesson is: we have to learn to deal with all our issues, learn to speak our truth, set clear boundaries and express our emotions in a healthy way.

Weight-problems are often a delayed emotional karma of things that happened in our youth. Some people have created a layer of fat around them to (metaphorically) protect them from getting attention they don't want. One example for this kind of shielding is a client of ours; let's call her Sybille.

Sybille was an unwanted 4th child and grew up in an emotionally and verbally abusive environment. Her siblings were the kind of shiny, successful people she would have loved to have been herself. The home environment was aggressive and ambitious. She was constantly being compared to her athletic, slim, successful siblings and felt she could never compete with their "perfection." Food was the only childhood pleasure she can remember having – it comforted her and numbed the pain of feeling unloved. Due to the years of programming of hearing how ugly, useless, unworthy, and unwanted she was, she simply gave up. She confessed that at times she wanted to end her life, as it didn't seem worth living. She did not believe she could ever step out of being a victim and have the strength to create a live she loved. She subconsciously used her fat to become invisible and prove how undesirable and unlovable she was. This old programming was still active in her when she came to see us and we helped her release that pattern in order for her to be able to lose weight and feel safe doing so.

Some people never liked their self-image and ate too much as a way of consoling themselves. Like Sybille, they felt it didn't matter any more: "they are unattractive anyway." Others were never taken seriously and being overweight gives them "more presence." These are just a few examples of the karmic reasons we put on weight and how our subconscious mind works.

Genetic karma

Then you have the karma of your genetic make up and you can have inherited the tendency to put on weight easily and have problems losing the weight or fat. Sometimes it is functional: if you are an Eskimo you may need the fat to protect you against the cold.

Past Life Karma (non linear time karma)

Two thirds of the world population believes in life after death. A big part believes in life after life, meaning we keep coming back (reincarnation). We cannot prove this scientifically and we cannot disprove it. But it may be true. So for this moment let's assume it is a possibility.

If you died from famine in a recent past life, you may take that past life memory of suffering from a lack of food with you into your current life. Your memory of having starved to death is so strong that you tend to overeat most of the time just to make sure you will never die of starvation again. You could struggle with being overweight all your life until that memory is healed. If in past lives you died of a disease that was linked to becoming very frail and fragile that has consequences too. In our experience, past lives can have an incredible effect on your eating habits, and the memory of those past lives have to be cleared for you to be free of that trauma. Your past life programs can be easily removed by someone who has been trained to do that.

Brain training is about changing the way you respond to life

In our training of the brain we pay attention to remove all past programming and we don't really care where that comes from, as it is not important. Compare it with a computer: when you have an expert clean up your computer from viruses, cookies and other stuff, you really don't care to know all the origins; you want two things:

1. Make sure that all negative impact is removed and
2. Be protected against it happening again.

That is exactly what we do with our Sleep Your Fat Away programming.

Why is this important?

The reason we explain this is because with Brain Training you can influence all these factors.

You can transform behaviors that do not support you, you can heal painful memories, you can let go of emotions and you change how you relate to food.

Brain Training boils down to you choosing to change the thought patterns and beliefs you have picked up from others. By changing them into patterns that support you and so allowing yourself to lead to a healthier, happier, and more successful life. The way you see yourself and give meaning to what happens to you determines your quality of life! By changing how you see yourself you are taking back control over you life instead of being a victim of past conditioning. In other words: it is about changing your negative karma into positive karma. We believe this is the way to go and have hundreds of client stories to prove this.

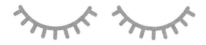

5

How to Beat the Tricks of the Food Industry

Before we get into training our brain, we need to go into why the food most of us are eating every day is making us sick and overweight. And how brain training is going to help teach your mind to love 'natural healthy foods'. Those super-foods that will help keep us slim, healthy, and happy.

The story of James

James came to see me with his mom; he was 17 and already very overweight! He was 5.11 and weighed 275 pounds; he had one of those big bellies that hung over his pants and also he was panting from the walk to my office. But the real reason he came to see me was because of his headaches and because was waking up at night, tired during the day, and as a result, was snoozing in class.

I checked his eating habits and on the surface it did not sound so bad at all, until we dug deeper. He started the morning with a famous brand of cereal with loads of milk. The good part of this was that it said to be fiber rich, the bad news: it was loaded with sugar. Then he drank his big glass of OJ (full of sugar) in the morning. 3 times a week he ate a good American breakfast: cheese omelet with sausage and grits. As a snack he had a fiber-sugar rich granola bar (also from a famous brand), he would eat 2 or 3 of those because there were so tiny and not filling. Lunch was either a big fat turkey sandwich with lots of turkey, mayonnaise and some sour gherkins (pickles) or a ham and cheese sandwich and a natural juice drink (filled with sugar). In the afternoon he would again have 2 or 3 granola bars and a cola drink (filled with sugar). For dinner they would have a carbohydrate, meat packed meal with some veggies on the side. Then before bed he would have chocolate drink and sometimes a snack. I had a nutritionist calculate the calories and we came close to 4000 calories a day. His sugar intake was sky-high and he was suffering from hypoglycemia and insulin resistance. The family had no idea that their diet based on the propaganda they were fed was killing them and making them fat. And guess what… the whole family was more on the obese side. At this rate James would be diabetic before the age of 21! His liver was weakened by the onslaught of sugar and chemicals from his food and this was causing his headache. It took 9 months to get him back to a natural weight and change his eating habits into healthy ones. His headaches were gone after 3 months on a new nutritional regimen without the chemicals of processed foods and he was sleeping progressively better as his weight was going down!

The food industry: making profit at all costs

The food industry has become a chemical producer of worthless products, which give us little nutritional value, destabilize our biochemistry, and make us hopelessly addicted to foods that are bad for us.

They invest billions into research to find out how to make us food and snack addicts. They employ the best brains money can buy to fool our brains into liking certain chemical compounds. Then they use clever advertisement tricks to hypnotize us into buying their concoctions.

We are fighting against a powerful conglomerate of greedy industries driven by the capitalistic worldview of making profit at all cost without respect for their customer. It is in the best interest of the food industry to get you addicted early on so you keep coming back for more. Great research goes into the marketing and packaging of products so we as consumers are lured into buying them. Even the way a supermarket exposes its products is based on psychology and science to get you to buy more than you need.

We are tricked to lose our instincts

As a human species we have lost contact with our natural instincts what to eat and when to eat. Our blood-sugar levels and chemical imbalances are created by refined carbohydrates and the other refined or processed foods we eat.

Our palate fools us; we fall in the trap of the food industry and eat more than is good for us or eat foods that are not good for our long-term health!

The best foods are the ones that are the least unprocessed and least chemically treated. The closer to nature, the better the food. That is how simple it is.

DNA: our cavemen genetics

Remember our antique bodies are not genetically adapted to deal with the chemical processed foods that have become our household staples. We live in modern times but we are physically not much evolved from the hunters we were not so long ago in this planet history. Genetically we are practically the same as our forefathers who roamed this planet for food and shelter.

Becoming fat is only one consequence of these genetically enhanced and chemically processed foods. The other karmic consequences of our processed foods are degeneration, arthritis, diabetes, premature aging, heart disease, and many other modern time physical problems.

Why you're fat and how you've been tricked into eating junk food

Marketers are paid a lot of money to get you to eat unhealthy food. And they're really good at their jobs.

There are these clever commercials with joyous young people munching on crispy potato chips or drinking a diet drink… or the billboard of the world famous athlete offering you a refreshing sip of an energy drink that you drove past on your way to work… and the magazine ad of a healthy looking family enjoying some pre fabricated meal that you read about at the dentist's office, etc.

On average we're exposed to nearly 3,000 marketing messages daily. Research shows that the images and associations these ads form within our minds eye are much more powerful than we realize. They influence our behavior and form a memory pattern that hides deep in our subconscious mind.

What's the deal?

"Any advertiser will tell you that successful marketing appeals to emotions and slips below the radar of critical thinking," says Marion Nestle, Ph.D., the author of the groundbreaking book, "Food Politics." "We are not supposed to notice advertising and we don't—unless we deliberately set out to look for it."

Anchors

Marketers want you to automatically associate their brand with happy feelings; they anchor a positive feeling to their products. They do this by linking their brand to basic human motivations—like accomplishments, fun activities, belonging, and self-fulfillment—to boost product sales.

Happiness, health, and playfulness sells

You watch them on TV and in magazine ads—the beautiful people, having fun; the sun is shining, perfectly toned bodies dance to well known pop tunes or jingles urging you to "enjoy life, the moment" and live "the lifestyle you dream of". They purposely suggest you not to think of the karmic consequences of your actions but instead focus on the instant gratification. And what's easier than getting a quick high from some chemical cocktail?

You know you're watching a phony commercial, but still you feel a little warm and excited. You even smile, as on a subconscious level your mind remembers a time when you were happy.

That's exactly how, for example, Coca-Cola, the company behind some really powerful commercials, wants you to feel. They unconsciously make you form an emotional attachment with their brand. The next time you're sipping a cola drink, you'll think of that commercial, the positive reward centers in your brain will light up, and you'll feel great.

Effective marketing makes you think you are in control

Effective marketing makes us *think* our reactions are completely rational: People try to sell us their products; we take that information for what it's worth, and then we think we make an informed decision. Research tells a different story. We believe we make rational choices when in reality we make highly emotional ones and rationalize them later.

The images and associations these ads form within our mind's eye are much more powerful than we think, many of them contain subtle psychological features that people don't understand or chose not to believe are there.

Get them while they're still young

Children are most receptive to marketing messages—their minds are like sponges, ready to soak up all information they receive. Marketers use this vulnerable time to develop "brand imprinting"—a term psychologists use to describe the process of encoding a particular brand in our brain's memory network through repeated brand name exposure.

The food industry spends in the US alone 11 billion annually to ensure we're putting our money where our mouth is. "Happy Meals" of McDonald's and all kinds of free toys is a great way to imprint that brand for life in the minds of our young ones.

Brand loyalty can begin as early as age 2—the age where children begin to recognize and develop a liking for familiar characters and can identify products in grocery aisles and request them by name.

Must have my happy meal

Enter "pester power," a term that refers to children's ability to nag their parents to buy advertised products, and you are buying stuff for your kids you want to protect them from. The "Happy Meals" often are linked to toys from popular movies to make them a 'must-have' for children and then there are the playgrounds where they can play after the happy meal… an ingenious package.

The brand imprints we gather as a child are often carried into adulthood. The alcohol and tobacco brand you're exposed to when younger are the ones you're more likely to try later.

A virus, just like with a computer, can infect your brain

The analogy we used before is the infestation of a computer with viruses and 'cookies' coming from use on the Internet. With our brain training we will clean your mind of all these implanted subconscious messages and conditioning that can often be worse than the faulty programming you have received from your parents. As opposed to a computer, your mind cannot be cleansed with one session. Just like the messages have been implanted by repeated exposure, the cleansing process involves the same. That is the big advantage of this programming over standard hypnosis and other therapies. You get to train your mind in your own time every night! The nightly brain training sessions as one of our biggest breakthroughs: it lets you use your sleep time (where your mind is completely open and does not filter the messages coming in) effectively. More on this subject in the chapter "Train your Brain and Sleep Yourself Slim."

Reclaim your brain

Today's manufacturers produce a wide range of hyper-palatable foods – full of sugar, fat and salt. These foods trick the reward center in our brain and make us want more of them. And we find these foods literally everywhere (at the register in your favorite coffee house, gas station…), are cheap and ready to go. As we get hooked to this type of food we are no longer attracted to natural foods like a bowl of berries or an apple, we rather go for a sugar laden energy/protein bar, pop-tart or muffin. And within the shortest time the reward center (which produces Dopamine – that body made drug that makes us feel great) in our brain is numbed into submission. It cannot handle so much over-stimulation and our brain literally changes to adapt. Recent studies funded by the National Institutes of Health have shown that the brain scans of food addicts show the same changes and damage as those of a cocaine user. The effects of this are that we need more and more of this food to get us the same fix and are constantly hungry.

Ways out of the addiction cycle

1. Become aware of what's going on. Don't allow anyone to subconsciously infiltrate your mind. You must be the one deciding what you want your brain to be programmed with. So don't have the TV running in the

background all day, pay attention to what the ads are trying to sell you (this can be a fun exercise and great learning experience!), don't believe everything that is said, read what's in the food you are eating and then decide what is best for you.

2. Don't trust the pretty labels on the front – read the ingredients on the back of the food you are eating! Remember that clever marketing knows exactly what to write on to a food to make you think it's good for you. Favorite words are "farm fresh, all natural" and hot ever since food intolerances have reared their head: "gluten free" or "fat free" – very often these products are filled to the brim with sugar. It's a simple rule of thumb: If you take something out of a natural food you have to replace it with something else to still taste nice.

3. Become a detector of quick fix foods and stop buying them! Step by step, wean yourself of the secret brain destroyers and retrain your palate to liking natural foods. You can repair the damage created in your brain. Every time you meditate and train your brain, you are actually strengthening brain cells and helping repair your brain. Our Sleep Your Fat Away daytime audios are the perfect helpers for this. Not only will you get into the habit of taking a Power-Break (which will enhance your productivity, heighten your awareness, spark your creativity and give you loads of energy), you will also be helping your brain recover and grow strong!

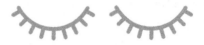

6

Shrink your Stomach and Lose Weight Effortlessly
with the Virtual Gastric Band

The real gastric band

In a surgical operation, requiring anesthesia, a band is placed like a collar around the top end of the stomach to create a small pouch. This pouch is the size of tennis ball and holds approximately ½ cup of food, whereas the typical stomach holds about 6 cups of food. When the gastric band patients eat, their pouch fills up quickly and the band slows down the passage of the food into the lower part of the stomach. As the upper part fills up, the stomach signals "**FULL**" to the brain (just like without a gastric band, but whilst in the past one had to fill up the whole stomach, now only the small pouch is filling up). This effect (the signal being sent to the brain after only eating ½ cup of food) helps the person to be hungry less often, feel full more quickly and for a longer period of time. Gastric band patients report eating much smaller portions and lose weight over time.

60

My mom and her gastric band

Roy: My mother had a real gastric band operation when she was about 65 years old. In the beginning very happy with her gastric band, she could no longer eat like she used to and had to chew more as she would get the feeling of something stuck in her throat if she swallowed too big of a bite without chewing. She soon discovered that she preferred soups to regular meals because those were easier to get down. Gradually and over time she got accustomed to eating smaller portions. What did not change were her cravings. She still craved chocolate and sweets and actually now that she was eating less, she start snacking more, sometimes even preferring to snack rather than eat proper meals. In the end the gastric band became useless, after initially losing some weight, she gained everything back over time and was back to square one. Being witness of my mom's experience with gastric band, I understood that the gastric band is just a symptomatic treatment and does not solve the real underlying problems. I am not saying that the same happens to all other gastric band patients, I am just stating that the gastric band does not tackle the complex of factors involved in weight-gain. That is why we made sure that in our "Sleep Your Fat Away" program we would address all angles of the problem and not only a smaller stomach size.

The real gastric band continued

Thousands of gastric band operations are performed on mostly obese patients every year. It is mainly applied to people who are severely overweight, facing obesity related health issues, have a history of obesity, are over 18 and not older than 60, and where all other methods of weight control have failed. Patients have to meet certain requirements to be considered candidates for this operation and many obese persons cannot have this operation due to the involved health risks and/or for financial reasons.

According to the American Society for Metabolic Bariatric Surgery, gastric band surgery is not an easy option for obesity sufferers. It is a drastic step, and carries the usual pain and risks of any major gastrointestinal surgical operation. Gastric band patients not only have to take on the risks of surgery, they also have to comply with the substantial lifelong dietary restrictions required for long-term success.

The alternative

Now what if you could have the positive effects of gastric band surgery without any negative side effects? This is where our brain training techniques come into action! In our Sleep Your Fat Away program, we use techniques used in hypnotherapy to retrain our client's subconscious mind into believing their stomach is significantly smaller, as if they've actually had gastric band surgery. Of course the user knows that they haven't had a surgical intervention, but due to the unique approach of reshaping the subconscious mind, their body and brain responds as though they have.

The revolution in weight loss and hypnosis

This new technique has increased the success rate from hypnosis from an average 35% to over 95%. The hypnotist Sheila Granger has clinically tested this in the UK and the tests have been repeated twice with the same results. In other words: hypnosis has proven to be as effective as surgery! Or: This hypnosis procedure has been tested scientifically to be as effective as the real procedure! Sheila was one of the first to start with this in England and has worked with thousands of overweight people and has been featured in popular English magazines many times. We had the pleasure of being taught by her and have modified the program to make it independent from a hypnotist. This way everyone can do this at home and afford to do so. And to make quite sure that we get the same (or even better) results than Sheila Granger, we added more powerful components to the program. It is our mission to help you end the misery of being overweight and we want this to be accessible to as many people as possible.

Your new best friend

Allow us to introduce your new friend and partner in weight loss: your virtual gastric band.

By having your virtual gastric band *"fitted in your subconscious mind"* you are receiving a wonderful help on your journey to the slim, healthy you. It stops you from over-eating while you learn to regain your natural responses to your body's signals. This makes it a lot easier for anyone to lose weight. You can compare it with an alcoholic who gets a treatment that when they drink they feel bad. The virtual gastric band has a similar effect it stops you from eating too much and this way you can start breaking the old patterns.

What does the virtual gastric band do?

Before you get the virtual gastric band, your stomach is about the size of a melon. It can expand to a very large melon, when you eat a lot and when not used to eating large amounts it can also shrink in size. When your stomach is full, you feel full. When you overeat, you can feel bloated and your stomach can feel painful. When you habitually overeat you stretch your stomach and you can eat, much more than you need without feeling too bad.

The virtual gastric band is as effective as the real gastric band because your body reacts to the implanted memory of having a gastric band procedure created in the sessions. Remember how we explained the way your subconscious mind works? It's like a child's mind, it takes everything very literally, and in Sleep Your Fat Away, we are using this effect to your benefit. Even though you consciously know very well that you have not had surgery, your subconscious mind will believe it has and react accordingly.

With the virtual gastric band you simply can't eat as much, you will feel full much sooner.

One of the things we like about this approach is that every overweight person can use this technique, no matter how young or old they are and what health restrictions they have. Just think what wonderful shifts we could help create in the growing epidemic of childhood obesity! If only we were already helping young children eat healthily by training their brains to listen to their bodies! We could be saving our society a lot of pain and money… Read more about the brain states and the correlated effects of childhood programming in the chapter "Eliminate Self-Sabotage and Become Your Best Friend."

The virtual gastric band: The preparation and installation

Just like with a real operation, you need to prepare! We want to achieve the maximum effect in all our techniques, which is why we created the first audio session of the program called "preparation for the virtual gastric band." This audio gets your brain ready for the actual installation of the band, heightens the excitement (just think how nervous you would be before the real operation!) and you listen to it for a week. Most people notice the effects of this audio and start eating less effortlessly. This way we mimic the real life situation where you know you are getting a gastric band before you have the actual operation. By doing this we make the subconscious installing of the virtual gastric band even more real!

In the second audio session called "Installing the virtual gastric band" you will be taken through the procedure in such a way that it will create an imagined memory that is more powerful than a real event. By the fact that it is relived at least 10 times in detail (second week), you are ingraining this memory in your brain. Your subconscious mind cannot tell the difference between an imagined operation and a real one. And by listening to this audio so often, it automatically gets stored in the depths of your subconscious memory banks. We have noticed this to be more powerful than just having one hypnosis session to install the virtual gastric band.

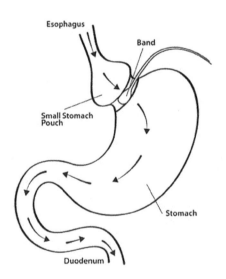

Now you feel the effects even stronger and your stomach will tell you when you have eaten enough to reach your goals. This is even better than a real surgery because with a 'real' surgical gastric band, you have to be aware and carry all the risks of surgery (complications, the risk of blood clots…).

The virtual gastric band offers you all the benefits without the negative side effects! Everything happens on a sub-conscious level and you have no negative side effects to worry about.

The two ways to get a virtual gastric band

One way is through a hypnosis session with a Sleep Your Fat Away weight loss expert or a hypnotist who understands the procedure; in personal sessions your expert will prepare and guide you through the process and be able to tackle unique personal issues. But as we stated before there are not many experts in the U.S. yet. This is why we also provide an expert training. We want to train as many therapists as possible so they can use this incredible technique in their practice! So if you are a coach or therapist yourself, we recommend you to take the special video training we created from a live seminar. We need more experts to help more people achieve their prerogative: a naturally slim body.

The second way is through the audio program we provide in our program on SleepYourFatAway.com. We have designed a specific "Virtual Gastric Band Session," where you are equipped with this splendid helper. All you need to do is relax and listen to this guided meditation. We will guide you through the procedure and your brain will do the rest. At last your subconscious mind is actively helping you rather than sabotaging you!

The effect is reinforced in our nightly Sleep Your Fat Away program. This allows your brain to adjust the virtual gastric band to fit your needs. You simply listen to the nightly recording (at a barely audible level in the background) whilst you sleep.

An alternative option is to start with our special guidelines and do it all by yourself at no extra costs. This program is also very effective and will help you to get back to the patterns of a naturally slim person. It requires a little bit more discipline but it can be done quite easily and is a great alternative to the dieting-fads that don't work in the long term. When we study the people who lost weight and kept if off, we discovered that they were not dieting but changed their lifestyle. And that is exactly what the guidelines will teach you.

So what we are saying is that even though the gastric band makes it much easier, it can also be done without that procedure if you wish to.

Michaela's experience

I have never meditated nor seen a hypnotist. So when I had my first sessions with Joy I was nervous and very skeptical. But I had tried and failed so many diets and couldn't shift the extra pounds I had gained after my two pregnancies that I was willing to try anything. In our second session I had my Virtual Gastric Band installed and I remember my thoughts at the beginning of the session. I could hear Joy's voice and thought "oh well this is relaxing and nice" but a part of me was worried about not being able to go deep enough…and that this stuff wouldn't work on me. I was so relieved when Joy gave me the suggestion of just having to relax, I think she even said "you don't need to go into trance, just play along – it's like a game". After that I just let go and it felt like listening to a story. I was surprised at the sensations and emotions I felt during the session, it was similar to watching a movie inside of my mind and I was having fun. I felt very aware of everything that was happening around me and felt totally in control. When we finished it was late afternoon and I drove home to cook dinner for my family. At dinnertime, I ate slowly and consciously and noticed (to my great amusement and surprise) how my family had also adopted my slower eating pace. We played the game of putting down our silverware in between bites and the kids started a competition as to who could eat slowest. My husband commented on how much more relaxed I seemed and what a fun atmosphere we were having at our table. We had more time to chat and listen to each other. Only then did I realize that I hadn't even eaten half of what was on my plate! And I felt really full and satisfied! This was certainly a first for me as I was usually the one finishing off not only my plate but also the kid's plates. I felt so proud of myself! And the best part is that it has been like that ever since! I feel far more in control and generally more relaxed about life at the same time. Even when the kids are having a tough day and things are stressful, I make a point of having a down time/me time and listening to the audios. In the meantime I love meditating and Joy's voice sends me into trance so quickly that I have a hard time staying awake. I have lost all the extra weight I gained with my boys; it happened to easily and effortlessly that I really couldn't say I suffered one day. And when my kids comment on how cool I look now, I feel like the Queen of the world!

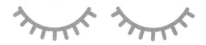

7

Why You Need to Sleep to Lose Weight

antasy writer Jim Butcher once wrote: "Sleep is God. Go worship." In this chapter we will explore why you want to follow his advice and how a lack of sleep can affect us more severely than we think.

On average we spend 36 percent of our life asleep, which means that if you live to 90, you have spent 32 years asleep. That is a lot of time and it is time we take our sleep seriously as it plays a vital role in keeping us physically and mentally healthy.

If we go back in time to the area of no electricity, our sleep was mainly regulated by the natural cycles of day and night. Once Edison made his ingenious invention of the light bulb, things started to change rapidly and so did our sleep patterns. Edison himself was even quoted saying "Sleep is a criminal waste of time..." and this quote gives us an idea of our general attitude towards sleep. On whole we think it's the least productive time of our lives and seek to get more and more crammed into the day; so shortening our time in bed to the max. We have continued to nip away at our nightly hours and on average sleep 1.5 hours less than we did in the 1950's. (In the 50's we were sleeping around 8 hours, today it's more like 6.5 hours.)

Actually, sleep is an incredibly important part of our biology, and neuroscientists are beginning to explain why we need to give our nightly hours more attention and value. Russell Foster, a British neuroscientist, explains the all-important link between the functionality of our brains and the amount of sleep we are getting. When we are asleep, our brains don't shut down. Actually some areas of the brain are more active during the sleep state than during the wake state.

Sleep doesn't arise from a single structure within the brain, but is to some extent a network property. Sleep arises from a whole raft of different interactions within the brain, and is also turned on and off through these interactions.

Why do we sleep?

There are many different ideas about why we sleep: from the more known restorative and regenerative effects, to more complex ones such as brain processing and memory consolidation. Foster: "What we know is that, if after you've tried to learn a task, and you sleep-deprive individuals, the ability to learn that task is smashed. So sleep and memory consolidation is also very important. However, it's not just the laying down of memory and recalling it. What's turned out to be really exciting is that our ability to come up with novel solutions to complex problems is hugely enhanced by a night of sleep. In fact, it's been estimated to give us a threefold advantage. Sleeping at night enhances our creativity. And what seems to be going on is that, in the brain, those neural and synaptic connections that are important, are linked and strengthened, while those that are less important tend to fade away and be less important."

Another research conducted by Maiken Nedergaard at the University of Rochester, claims our brains are busy in a clean-up process at night. "I think we have discovered why we sleep," Nedergaard said. "We sleep to clean our brains." Through a series of experiments on mice, the researchers showed that during sleep, cerebral spinal fluid is pumped around the brain, and flushes out waste products like a biological dishwasher. This process is more active during sleep because it takes too much energy to pump fluid around the brain when awake. The process helps to remove the molecular debris that brain cells churn out as part of their natural activity, along with toxic proteins, which can lead to dementia when they build up in the brain, the researchers say.

Foster concludes his studies of human sleep and it's effects on the brain with: "Sleep is not an indulgence. It's not some sort of thing that we can take on board rather casually. I think that sleep was once likened to an upgrade from economy to business class... (I think) It's not even an upgrade from economy to first class. The critical thing to realize is that if you don't sleep, you don't fly. Essentially, you never get there, and what's extraordinary about much of our society these days is that we are desperately sleep-deprived."

What happens when we are sleep deprived?

Our society as a whole is not getting enough sleep. And some parts are suffering more than others: shift workers (their biological clock is totally out of balance and they, on the whole, get only 5 hours of nightly rest), frequent flyers suffering from jet lag, teenagers (they need 9 hours to function properly and are getting around 7 hours) and the huge group of chronically stressed people working long hours and juggling their career and private lives.

The danger of micro-sleeps

When our brain gets over-tired it has a natural response, which is to make you fall asleep for a few seconds, similar to a reboot of a computer system. This involuntary falling asleep can be sort of somewhat embarrassing, but they can also be deadly. It's been estimated that 31 percent of drivers fall asleep at the wheel at least once in their life. In the U.S. an estimated 100,000 accidents on the freeway have been associated with tiredness, loss of vigilance, and falling asleep.

Lack of sleep makes you fat

So when you lack sleep, you tend to get mores stressed, have poor memory, are less creative, suffer from increased impulsiveness, your immune system suffers, you have a higher risk of suffering from diabetes or a heart attack (and even cancer, as shown in studies of shift workers) and have overall poor judgment. But did you know that a lack of sleep also triggers unhealthy nutritional choices?

If you are a tired brain, the brain craves substances to wake it up: Stimulants like caffeine, alcohol, nicotine, and sugar. You will also find yourself craving more refined carbohydrates when you are tired.

If you sleep around about five hours or less every night, then you have a 50 percent likelihood of being obese. The lack of sleep raises the release of the hormone ghrelin, the hunger hormone. Ghrelin in the brain triggers the craving for carbohydrates and particularly sugars. So there's a link between tiredness and the metabolic predisposition for weight gain. Also the longer you are awake the more you tend to snack and consume in calories!

Out best tips for getting a good night's sleep

1. Turn your bedroom into a sanctuary and sleep haven
2. Make it as dark as you can
3. Keep it slightly cool
4. Reduce your amount of light exposure at least half an hour before you go to bed. Light keeps your brain awake and will delay sleep. Turn off the TV. Turn off mobile phones. Turn off computers. Turn off all of those things that are also going to excite the brain.
5. Avoid caffeine late in the day, ideally starting after lunch.
6. Don't indulge in high sugary foods and drinks before bed.
7. Do eat foods containing tryptophan, the natural sleep inducer, such as:
   - Beans
   - Whole grains, including rice
   - Lentils
   - Chickpeas
   - Hazelnuts
   - Peanuts
   - Eggs
   - Sunflower seeds
   - Sesame seeds
   - Miso (fermented soy beans)

- Unsweetened soy milk
- Dairy products (if you can tolerate dairy)

Drink a relaxing herbal tea like Chamomile, Valerian, Lavender, and St. John's Wart ...and only occasionally resort to red wine.

The benefits of a good night's sleep

If you are getting enough sleep you will be rewarded with

- Increased concentration and attention
- Enhanced decision-making
- Lower stress levels
- Less anger flares and impulsiveness
- Lower tendency to drink and take drugs
- Less cravings for sugary foods
- Reduced your mood swings
- More creativity
- Better social skills
- Radiant health
- Easy weight loss and being able to keep a healthy weight effortlessly!

Optimize your sleep!

So now we know that getting enough sleep is crucial to high energy levels, overall well being, mental and emotional sanity and a healthy weight... how can we optimize the time we spend snuggled up in bed?

Until we have discovered healthy options for reducing our sleep time, we feel it's best to use our sleep time effectively. So what if you could train your brain at night and without any effort?

Well, that's exactly where our Brain Trainings come in. We have developed a system, which makes the most of our natural brain states during sleep.

Read more about this ingenious, effective, and easy to apply method in the chapter: Train Your Brain and Sleep Yourself Slim.

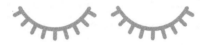

8

Train Your Brain and Sleep Yourself Slim

This program is unique and different from the other programs available.

The secret ingredients

What makes this program so powerful is the combination of the reinforcement of the virtual gastric band effect and training the brain by installing the new habits of naturally slim people, so the program becomes so easy to follow. We especially like the fact that for most people this program is totally effortless and they are making real life style changes.

Ellen Noor: it feels like cheating

Here is a testimonial of Ellen Noor, a kindergarten teacher in Holland. She was interviewed in a popular Dutch magazine and said:

After trying every type of diet I start feeling like a hopeless case. I gained over 30 kilos, 10 kilo for every pregnancy and it was incredible hard for me to lose weight. I don't have the discipline to see a diet through to the end and after a few setbacks I give up. Then I get desperate again when my weight goes up and I start the next one. The best so far was the carbohydrate free diet, but after awhile it gets boring and I start losing track. Now I have lost over 24 kilos on the audio program of the virtual gastric band. First of all I never got so far on any weight loss program before! When people compliment me about my weight loss, I tell them that it was so easy that I feel like cheating because I know how difficult it is to lose weight! For me it is like child's play, I put my audio on before going to sleep and that is it! I just notice the changes in my daily life. I feel less hungry, have less mood swings, like walking more. I feel better about myself, I notice I feel more playful and notice myself humming songs, I genuinely feel happy, and as a bonus I lost weight. It is a miracle!

This is just one of the many testimonials we have and they are all stating very similar experiences! Because the programming is not based on willpower and focuses on changing the subconscious programming, it doesn't feel like you are trying to lose weight. It is just being conscious of what you do without forcing anything!

Imitating real life

In order to install a new memory of an imaginary event, which appears to be more real for the body than a real event, we have pioneered a few interesting new hypnotic approaches.

1. The set up is as staged in such a way that the mind is prepared for the installation of the gastric band. For example if you are going to have a surgical procedure such as the gastric band, you know this some time before the event. We created a session for you listen to for a week before the procedure, to go through that natural sequence of anticipation and preparation like you would before a regular surgery.

This session creates a tension in your body and it will enhance the implementation of the memory!

2. Then we take you through the procedure with real hospital sounds and the imagining of smells and other factors of a hospital. This is done in such a way that for the subconscious mind the created memory is accurate and realistic. Listening to the recording of the virtual gastric band at least 10 times creates a very vivid recall. The result being that this memory is so powerful; it evokes strong reactions at the level of neurotransmitters in the brain. The feelings created by the repetition of the imagined scenario become real even though the event is not real. The subconscious mind accepts these images and fills in the blanks to make it complete.

3. Reinforcement: repetition is very important. It creates a process in the brain that will result in what are called neuro-synapses. This is especially important when dealing with the installation of new "good" habits: in the program you are guided to imagine already having these new power-habits and because of this, your brain creates the synapses like it would if you already had these habits. In real life you can then experience the habit as being a natural part of your life. The synapses result in what is called an autopilot, which eliminates the need to rely on will power. It becomes a new habit that is installed at the neurological level.

Here an example to make this approach even clearer to you: Remember how you first learn how to drive a car? At the beginning you had to consciously think of all the separate steps like turning the key, fastening the seat belt, putting the gears into drive, pressing down on to the accelerator, checking your mirrors, etc. We call this being consciously incompetent. You have to think about it. After practicing for a while you were quickly able to do all of these steps in automatic mode – you became unconsciously competent. And that is where we want you to go when it comes to eating healthily. Brain Training will help you achieve this desired state in a much faster way than if you were to do so on pure willpower.

Training your brain while you sleep

Sleep Programming is officially more powerful than hypnosis. It's recently been proven by the San Diego University and is used daily by the US Government to help train new military recruits. The new recruits get positive affirmations to listen to during the night and they become more self-assured, can manage their fears better, and are ready to go on dangerous missions much faster.

Sleep programming is a technique of feeding powerful suggestions to your mind while you sleep, reprogramming your thoughts at the deepest possible level. There are programs that help you learn a foreign language easily and quickly and to get a better grasp on the grammar, just by subconsciously listening while you sleep.

The ultimate help in weight loss

"Sleep Your Fat Away" is an extraordinarily powerful audio experience that will super-charge and train your brain to positively change your most basic beliefs and habits in regards to eating, food health and happiness at the level where it matters most: your deep subconscious mind. And it does it all while you enjoy a calm, restful sleep!

Sleep programming has been proven highly effective for thousands of people over many years, and Roy Martina M.D. is one of Europe's most renowned and respected holistic doctors, who has been using sleep programming for many years.

Roy: As you have read in the introduction, I started very young with sleep programming. Once I became a medical doctor and did not have to study for exams any longer, I stopped with that habit and started playing music instead during the night. I was reminded of the concept again when I saw a German executive diagnosed with cancer, which had metastized in his liver and bones. He was given only 3 months to live. He looked pale and greyish from the chemotherapy and was emaciated. A student referred him to me and I saw him during the lunch break of a workshop in Ebenhausen, (S-Germany). I gave him 3 things to do: change his diet to alkalinize his blood, visualize himself being healthy and happy again and to listen to a CD (from our Omega Healing series, called: "Anti Cancer"). This CD was created to train the brain to strengthen the immune system. I said because you have only a 3 months prognosis, I would listen to this at least 6 times a day and even put it on repeat during the night. It is not created for listening during the sleep but I strongly recommend it so you can turn this situation around. I saw him one year later and he was a totally changed man. The scan had revealed him as completely healed and he came back to thank me. His words were: "I know your voice better than my wife's and you saved my life! I have listened to you for an average of 12 hours a day. You gave me hope and strength, especially during the night. Right from the first day I could relax better during my sleep and I woke up every day refreshed and feeling better! Thank you."

That is when I understood that night programming could be used for healing and we started to play with it ourselves first and immediately noticed changes and deeper sleep.

Joy: We record sleep programs for each other and our kids depending on what every one of is working on. The kids take part in determining what they want in their sleep program and have great results with it. Our youngest child, Grace, is 4 years old and she insists on having her audio on all night. She grew up with sleep programming and we are delighted to see how healthy, smart, lively, and loving she is. We have noticed so many positive effects and changes in all of us since we do brain training at night that we have enough stories to fill another book. And we are working on creating a whole series of audios so that you can all take part in this great way of self-empowerment.

Her kindergarten teacher, Courtney, who baby-sat Grace for a week while we were on a business trip said: "I was so impressed that Grace wanted to listen to those audio sessions. So I also listened and it felt so good that I want to have them for myself! I believe all children should be listening to such positive messages during the night!"

Have your personal therapist sit at your bedside all night!

"Sleep Your Fat Away" is a collection of uniquely powerful strategies and is the culmination of 30 years of research and testing. They will work for you … even if

your conscious mind is skeptic. We like comparing the approach to having your personal therapist you trust and feel comfortable with, sit at your bedside every night, giving you positive affirmations; helping you build strong, empowering beliefs and letting go of old traumas.

Why is this different from other sleep programs?

1. The mistake many producers of sleep CD's make, even those that call their programs "sleep programming," is that they make 45-60 minutes recording and advise you to put that recording on repeat. This totally ignores the natural sleep rhythms of the body and can create fatigue or sleep deprivation in some sensitive people. If you are using these programs and waking up tired, then it is not working for you and you might want to try a new improved version. Another reason for not sleeping well with a nightly audio is that the volume is too loud and so disturbing you to get into a deeply relaxed state.

Important note:

Remember to have your nightly brain training on at a barely audible level! And you do NOT need to sleep with earphones – just have it running in the background and go to sleep. Your subconscious mind is always wide-awake and will get all the information it needs to help you lose weight!

2. Most of the programs on the market do not use the natural patterns of brainwaves during the sleep to their advantage. By knowing about the dream patterns one can use the dreams to help with the weight-loss by suggesting that the person will dream of losing weight and reach the desired weight. We call this proprietary technique Dream-Integration. This is very powerful and one of the great innovations we have created!

3. Most programs only give positive suggestions and have not incorporated techniques to neutralize the traumatic experiences of the past and that may become a problem for emotional eaters.

4. During sleep is an ideal time to give suggestions to increase the metabolism and burn more fat. This helps a lot for people who have done many diets and have a slow metabolism.

Our unique system

The duration

Our Sleep Your Fat Away sleep programming is much longer than normal guided meditations and consists of 10 unique components. Including setting the intention while still in alpha waves for the night (this is the phase you are automatically in when you are slipping off into sleep but still consciously aware of your surroundings), followed by the 5 rules so find it very easy to follow them during the day. By always setting your intention, you keep the subconscious mind focused on your goals and that way the program is 100% specific for your personal wishes and desires.

Specially designed brainwave technology

Neurologically stimulating sounds are used to induce dreamtime at night. These help create lucid dreaming about being slim, healthy, and happy with special white noise and with what is called binaural sounds.

Your mind will always be in a receptive state for the messages, thanks to the "binaural beat" and "monaural beat" brainwave technology used subliminally under the pink noise of this recording. This is EXTREMELY POTENT, and works with or without headphones!

High-speed subliminals

The subconscious mind picks up much more than the conscious mind! Furthermore the subconscious mind never sleeps. And we make use of this effect in the nightly brain training. We introduce the positive affirmations on a subliminal level for a deeper absorption; they are sped up to 3x times the normal speed. Subliminal means that the conscious mind cannot hear them, only the subconscious mind can. This improves the integration of the positive affirmations and speeds up the programming as the conscious mind is busy...sleeping!

Dream integration

Here we stimulate lucid dreaming with anchoring, pink noise and subliminals. The brain is conditioned to have happy dreams about already being thin, creating a sub-reality in the mind where the goals have already been met. This creates a neurological 3 dimensional template of experience that will stimulate the autonomous nervous system to follow in real life. This also means that you automatically create the experience of how it is to be naturally slim. This memory becomes so real that the body will follow and create it for you. You create what you see and imagine!

Right brain activation with metaphorical language

The right brain reacts to imagination and metaphorical language. This part of the programming helps to tap into the inner child aspect of our personality, create a new approach to release, let go of emotions and heal traumatic past events without any suffering. It is the most important part of the programming to work on the root cause of the weight gain. This is especially important for emotional eaters and compulsive eating disorders.

Reinforcement during the day

Subliminal programming

During the day there are audio-sessions you can put on in the background, they are subliminal. The conscious mind can only hear the music but not the words. And that is exactly what we want! This way your conscious mind cannot get in the way and challenge the positive affirmations. It will "allow" the positive, weight loss inducing and life transforming beliefs into your subconscious mind, which is where we want them to take roots. This will reinforce the sleep programming and keep you in a happy, energetic state. This is very important because some old programming is very strong (just think how long you have been thinking and re-thinking those limiting beliefs and negative thoughts!) and your conscious mind can interfere with the suggestions. Subliminal messaging is a way to bypass the critical mind and get the messages into the subconscious.

Emotional balancing

One of the things we have to learn to deal with, are our emotional patterns. All too often we are raised with the belief that we have no control over emotions and so have only 2 options:

- Express them and deal with the exterior consequences (the reactions of our environment to our emotional outburst)
- Suppress them and deal with the inner consequences (build of emotional charge resulting in disease and stress)

Part of our mission and passion is to show you that this is not true. You need not become a victim of your emotional state; instead you can learn to claim your power back by balancing your emotions without the stress.

We have created some powerful techniques to help transform emotions within minutes, so you can go from a stressful to a happy state.

Transforming does not mean suppressing, in the contrary: it is about feeling the emotion, acknowledging it, dealing with it rapidly and stepping back into your power. Most emotional patterns are conditioned responses coming from our youth and are completely useless. We have made special videos to train you how to easily deal with and manage your emotions. In these videos we demonstrate acupressure points to deal with stress, emotional hunger and emotions. You can learn more about this in the best selling book by Dr. Roy Martina: Emotional Balance (Hay House Publishing).

Conscious reinforcement:
Your Time Out session – a gift to all our readers!

We also give you a short recording (a power break) that you can put on your smart phone and listen to regularly, this will motivate you and inspire you to stay on your path.

This way you go fast and effortlessly and before you know it you are a fat burning machine.

As a reader of this book you can download Your Time Out/Power Break session for free here: www.sleepyourfataway.com. It is our gift to you so you can get a taste for what our program sounds like and try it out at no risk.

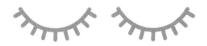

9 Eliminate Self-Sabotage and Become Your Best Friend

This might be the most important chapter of the whole book! Self love is the foundation of a happy and fulfilled life – and an essential part of any successful life style change – especially when it comes to weight loss. In this chapter we will explore how the way we see ourselves, determines how we treat ourselves and show you why it is crucial to become your number one fan if you want to become a naturally slim person. We will also share some simple and effective, practical practices to help you fall in love with yourself.

Brain waves and childhood programming

Show me your childhood, your parents, your peers and I will tell you who you think you are. Before you start getting all defensive because you think we are out to bash parents and point angry fingers at the your loved ones, relax. We are not in the blaming business. Rather we would like to show you

- How our childhood experiences form our belief systems
- That you are not the calm, rational decider you might think you are
- And that you have no idea who you really are and have just accepted other people's opinions about you.

What does a baby think?

Let's go back in time and for a moment imagine being that sweet little, defenseless baby. And let me tell you something about a baby's state of brain.

Fact is: The more relaxed your brain waves are, the easier it is for information to get into your head and literally program your mind.

What waves are my brain making?

Lets first look into the different brainwaves. There are 4 brainwave states we go through on a daily basis.

- Beta
- Alpha
- Theta
- Delta

When we are in <u>beta</u> we are conscious and our critical faculty protects our subconscious mind. We filter what we perceive and make up opinions and react based on our beliefs or emotions.

In <u>alpha</u> we are more relaxed and less critical, we are much more willing to see a bigger picture and are no longer governed by our critical mind. We are more open to new ideas, suggestions and are far more creative.

In <u>theta</u> we are deeply relaxed and very open, we have a hard time filtering information and start accepting much more at face value. We only resist what goes against our morals and deep beliefs. In this state we can change most of our beliefs about ourselves and accept more empowering beliefs. We are accustomed to go into sleep in this slow brain-activity.

<u>Delta</u> is our dream state and integration state, we here process the information we pick up during the day and also process our emotions.

Lets go back to babies

Now up to the age of 2 years, a baby's brainwaves are in the delta state most of the time. This is a deeply relaxed state that as a grown up you go into when you are fast asleep and will find virtually impossible to stay awake in. From the age of about 2-7 years of age our brain waves are predominantly in theta – still a very relaxed state and as grown up we aim to get into this state when we are experienced in meditation or are asleep at night. This means that as small children nearly everything we hear, see, and experience goes straight into that massive database of our subconscious mind and stays there for future reference.

Now picture this cute little baby or small child in it's daily surroundings. See it being cuddled by the mum or dad, hearing lullabies, listening, and watching all the things that go on every day in a home. There are good days and bad days. Sometimes parents are having a tough time, are tired or angry, and might have arguments to solve; on other days things are peaceful and loving. Think of your own childhood! I am sure you can also remember quite a wide scope of random elements, situations and happenings.

Sometimes you were reprimanded by your parents (in a more or less constructive manner) or told off at school. You maybe watched TV (or it was running in the background – think of the millions of adverts you heard subliminally!); listened to the radio, to adults' conversations (or fights) and faced arguments with your peers. Maybe you had a grandparent tell you the facts of life or give you their cents of wisdom. It's usually a kaleidoscope of memories you have stored within you – and unfortunately not all of it is helpful and empowering. Adding to the information we are consciously aware of and have access to (approximately 20%), the majority of data is stored at an unconscious or subconscious level.

The main programming of our brains happens before we hit age 7, as this is the time when we are most open to suggestions, information, and impressions. You see at that pre 7-age period and in those very relaxed brain states we are like sponges. At that age period we store *without* filter – hence the sweet naiveté of young children. As kids we are totally dependent on what others tell us how life works. As humans we learn by experience and only have our memory banks of experiences to go by when we make choices. (We like to think of ourselves as these very evolved, wise, and rational beings, who make intelligent, rational choices. But actually we make very emotional choices based upon our past experiences and then rationalize these afterwards… but that's another book.)

And you can imagine that by the time we are adults, we have a huge amount of data stored subconsciously within us. And this data also forms our self-image. Subconscious means under our conscious access level, you consciously have no access to these memories, only some memorable moments remain—mostly traumatic or happy experiences, or memories anchored to pictures or stories.

By the time we are 16 we have heard on average around 12,000 times who we are and who we are not; what we should do and what not; what we are good at and what not – and when we are so say mature we actually believe the stuff we were told and think this is who we are, because those messages have formed a matrix sub-reality that governs our perceived reality in the now.

What does your self-image have to do with being fat?

More than you think! In our practice with 1000s of overweight clients we have discovered some consistent patterns. One of them is that most overweight people lack self love, self worth and have a strong negative self-image. In other words: they don't like themselves much, do not believe they are worthy of love, success, a good life and are very harsh critics of themselves.

Karin's story

Karin was the child of an alcohol addicted, abusive father, and a meek mother. As a girl she learn fast that in order to get through childhood she had to become "invisible." Coming home was like Russian roulette. She never knew what state her dad would be in and how toxic the atmosphere would be. When dad was having a good day, he would be very kind and they'd have fun as a family. But on the bad days it was like walking a minefield. Karin had to watch her step, be as "good" as she possible could and keep out of his way. He would be irritable, aggressive, and abusive – verbally and physically. Karin was powerless to his transgressions and had to endure many a painful situation. He was particularly good at telling her how useless, ugly, and stupid she was. After a time, she learnt to numb herself against the verbal attacks. Eating was one of the ways she found to console and comfort herself – at least that was a "safe" occupation. When Karin hit puberty she was already overweight and she faced more verbal onslaught from her peers at school. When we first met her, our first thought was "she is wearing an armor of fat." Everything about this young woman screamed "I hate myself." She said herself that she found herself unattractive and unworthy of love. When we started working with her, she started remembering all the careless, negative comments she had been confronted with a kid. Once she realized that she did not have to hold on to these false, limiting beliefs about herself and could instead integrate empowering beliefs, things changed fast. She was able to let go of the painful, past experiences and forgive. She no longer identified with what others had told her who and how she was. Karin developed a new self image based on what she wanted to achieve in life and who she wanted to be. In a few personal coaching sessions, we helped her create a new script for herself and with the help of our "Sleep Your Fat Away" program she completely reprogrammed the way she saw herself, eliminated her negative thoughts about herself *and* lost weight. I remember the day she phoned us to say: "You know, I think I am getting a glimpse of what it is like to love myself!" When we saw Karin again after 6 months she had dropped 25 pounds in weight. And even more importantly: instead of the insecure, unhappy young lady struggling with life, we saw a confident, radiant young woman who believed in herself and was working toward her goals.

If you believe you will fail or succeed – both is true

It's up to you to decide what you want to go for. Do you want to continue seeing yourself as a failure and stay a victim of your inner sabotage? Or are you ready to take responsibility for what you have created for yourself? And yes, you read right: YOU created whatever you are facing. Whether we like it or not: our "outer" life represents a mirror of our inner life. So if you don't like what you are seeing, it's time to start asking yourself a potentially life changing question:

What do I need to stop doing?

Your thoughts become your beliefs, your beliefs become your habits, and actions and these determine your character and your destiny. You can be your greatest fan or enemy – make a guess what attitude will support your goals most.

What destiny would you like to create for yourself? And what part of you is stopping you from doing just that? What are your most frequent negative thoughts? What does your negative self talk sound like? What self-destructive habits do you indulge in?

Your date with yourself

Let's get practical and help you with your personal fan club. Do yourself the favor and put at least one of these steps into action now. Reading "How To's" is good; putting them into practice is much, much better.

Step one: Listen

Before we can start focusing on what you want, you need to assess your status quo and find out where you are now. There is no need to go into a rant about yourself but you do need to be honest and take over full responsibility for what is.

Take a few minutes right now to sit in silence, close your eyes and ask yourself: what do you need to stop doing and thinking?

Make a note of the answer you receive.

Step two: Accept what is

However much you dislike what you are seeing and realizing about yourself now: this is where you are now. And as frustrating or upsetting this situation may be for you, you have in this very moment also made the first and essential step towards change. You have realized, recognized, and accepted what is. So many don't even get this far. They are so busy denying and suppressing what they don't want that they become blind and numb. You are different; you are making a change – be proud of yourself!

Sam's story

Sam (54) had been overweight since he was 12 years old. His story was one of physical and sexual abuse by a neighbor, since the age of 7. He had threatened that he would kill him if he told his parents. He became introverted, depressed and started eating his emotions away since the age of 8. He was now married but traumatized and had problems with intimacy even though his wife was a kind and loving person. He did not have the money for personal sessions and chose to do a trial with "Sleep Your Fat Away" program. This experience totally transformed his life within 4 weeks; not only did he lose weight but his relationship changed. He was able to finally free himself of the past trauma and let go of the guilt he had carried with him all those years. He no longer felt like a victim and become the person he wanted to be. For him, forgiving his abuser was the biggest breakthrough.

Acceptance means letting go of judgments and choosing for freedom

Take a few deep breaths, close your eyes and accept. Be with what is for a few minutes. Feel how liberating realization can be. Don't judge yourself, don't beat yourself up. Instead be gentle, kind and compassionate towards yourself. By becoming aware of being a neutral observer of yourself, you are already making a shift. Maybe you would like to say something like this to yourself (we would normally call it "a prayer" as we are great believers in the power of prayer. But to make this book as accessible as possible for many, we refrain from using religious sounding words. Because this book and concept is not about religion, it is about awakening a power/force that resides within every one of us!)

I forgive myself for all the mistakes and bad choices I made in the past. I at that time did not know better and now I do.

Thank you, Higher Self/Divine Power/God/Universe (chose the word you feel comfortable with) for making me aware of what I am doing to myself. I know that whatever is, is a blessing and gift. For through this situation I can access my true potential and claim my power back. I have everything in me to make the changes I need to make. I am grateful for all the blessings in my life and for being me. From now on I promise myself to honor the Divine in me and take control of my life.

Step 3: Time for a change!

Now we can get busy. Here's a quick way to actively reprogram your self-image and install some powerful new beliefs. Do this exercise at least twice a day, preferably in front of you vision board (see the references at the end of the book for tips on creating a vision board)

1). Do the "Switch" and neutralize your limiting, negative beliefs.

This step is crucial to trick your brain out of the sabotage mode. Just affirming what you'd like to believe—repeating positive affirmations— unfortunately does not work. Positive affirmations alone make your mind immediately go into sabotage mode and rebel…and all your well-meant work is for nothing. Actually your system gets really stressed by repeating what it thinks is nonsense all the time.

The secret is to successful distract the conscious mind by doing the switch (you have to focus on that movement in order not to whack yourself) and by stating "I love myself even if…" you are acknowledging the fact that you don't like yourself, think your fat and ugly etc. and so your conscious mind doesn't have to start a rebellion and will accept the new beliefs, which you are installing in step 2. Additionally The Switch stimulates many acupressure points in your hands and activates the corresponding organs in your body. It's also a quick way to give you an energy boost and alleviate tension headaches.

How to do "The Switch"

Like a Karate move, hit your left fist into your right open palm and then alternate (so hit your right fist into your left open palm) and do it as fast as you can. And while you are doing this movement you say:

"I love and accept myself even if I don't like myself and cannot let go of my negative self image and I love and accept myself if I now choose to love myself just the way I am."

You can make this statement very personal and specific for what you are feeling. If you are having a bad day and feel ugly/fat/unworthy you could say:

"I love and accept myself even if I think I am ugly, fat and unworthy and I love and accept myself if I now let go of those beliefs and choose to think of myself as beautiful, slim and worthy of the best that life has to offer."

Watch this short clip on our YouTube channel to see how the Switch goes.

2). Install your new beliefs with the Crown-Heart-Chakra Integration (CHI)

This "magical" movement balances your energy-centers (also known as Chakras) and allows you to step out of your head and connect to your heart. By you having to focus on the movement plus the effect this has on your energy centers, it allows your brain to accept the positive affirmations more easily. It's actually as if your conscious mind gets out of the way and the door to your subconscious mind opens up.

How to do the CHI

Standing or sitting upright, with one hand gently tap the air above your head (your crown chakra) and then move down to the space in front of your heart (your heart chakra) and tap the air there. Then go up to your crown chakra again and keep moving up and down while you repeat your affirmations. You can watch a short clip on www.sleepyourfataway.com to see how the CHI goes.

Below please find some powerful affirmations to work with. Pick the ones that resonate most strongly with you. Start with a maximum of 5. Work with those for a month and then move on to the next set. You can reinforce the affirmations by writing them out on a flashcard, pin them next to your mirror, stick them to the dashboard of your car...the more often you see them and repeat them, the better!

3). Your affirmations for a healthy body image and weight loss

I love and respect myself just the way I am.

I forgive myself for making bad choices and know that I now have the power to make wise choices, which reflect my self-love.

Today I chose to love and honor my body fully, deeply and joyfully.

I am a beautiful divine being and I am on my path to being slim and healthy.

I enjoy eating healthy foods.

Every day I am getting closer to my goal of losing xxx pounds of fat and becoming a healthy, slim, and happy person.

Every night I sleep my fat away; I am a fat burning machine.

I trust my body's wisdom and I enjoy listening to my body's needs.

My body is the home of my soul and I enjoy looking after it.

I am growing more beautiful and radiant every day.

I choose to see the divine perfection in every cell of my body.

As I love myself, I allow others to love me too.

I love the way I feel when I take good care of myself.

Today my own well being is my top priority.

I believe in myself and know that I deserve the best that life has to offer.

The more I love myself the more love I have to share.

I am a role model for health and well being.

Every day I get better at looking after myself and loving all parts of myself.

I am safe, I am loved, I am love, I am worthy, I am courageous, I am determined, I am at peace, I am grateful, I am forgiving, I am kind, I am generous, I am successful, I am healthy, I am happy, I am wise, I am unstoppable.

Our free gift for you – start training your brain today!

We have made a special brain training audio (called "Subliminal Brain Training") for you, where these affirmations are implemented in a subliminal recording. You can find these on our website www.sleepyourfataway.com. The great thing about this audio format is that you can have it running in the background while you work and play. All you will consciously hear is some relaxing music – but your subconscious mind is being bombarded with positive affirmations and new beliefs and so in time you are equipped with a more empowering self-image automatically. And that will affect all areas of your life in a magical, positive way!

3 Keys to Becoming Your Greatest Fan

Stop worrying!

Worrying is a total waste of energy (and I know what I am talking about! I used to spend a lot of time worrying about possible future events that never came.)

Think of how much more pleasant your thoughts and so days will become when you start thinking about what you actually want instead of focusing on your fears. My mum always says: "We will cross that bridge when it comes!" And how right she is. Have trust in yourself and that higher power which created you and all that is. You have everything in you to be able to deal with whatever happens. What's the point in mentally preparing for disasters that most of the times don't happen anyway? And if disaster does strike, you will deal with it then. In the meantime give up your addiction to the fear based thoughts and start enjoying life.

Forgive

Holding grudges keeps you locked in the past. It prevents you from moving on and creating your desired life. Being angry with someone who did you wrong hurts you, not the other. Forgiving is what you need to do for yourself to be free. Forgiveness is not about agreeing with the other; it is about letting go of the toxic emotions and energy you are carrying around with you. Being angry, holding grudges and being resentful stresses your system and eventually makes you sick. We have seen too many resentful, angry people struggle with back pain and cancer – don't make that mistake and start forgiving today. Who or what is worth killing yourself for? Wouldn't you rather be having fun in life and manifest your heart's desires?

The How To De-link and Forgive Practice

1. The Switch

Like a Karate move, hit your fist into your open palm – alternate and do it as fast as you can. And you say:

"I love and accept myself even if I cannot let go of this pain/past incident/ anger/resentment/guilt/judgment etc. and I love and accept myself if I now choose to completely let go of this and step into my power of forgiveness.

2. Crown-Heart-Chakra & Forgiveness

Tapping the air above your head and in front of your heart (and continuously moving back and forth), you say (whilst imagining that person or situation in front of your mind's eye):

"I claim my power back and I give you your power back.
I claim my freedom back and I give you your freedom back.
I claim back what's mine and I give you what's yours.
I forgive you for all the pain and suffering you caused me and I ask you for forgiveness for all the pain and suffering I have caused you.
The past remains in the past. I now cut the cords. Only love can connect us.
I wish you well, just as I wish myself well."

If you like working with Angels and Ascended masters, you can additionally ask Archangel Michael for help, to cut the links with his flaming sword and you can call upon the Ascended Master Saint Germain to light his ultraviolet flame and burn the karma between you.

4. End with a prayer of gratitude
Be grateful for the lessons you learn through this incident and meditate on how this helped you, made you stronger/wiser/more loving.
You are done forgiving and delinking when you can wish upon the other what you wish for yourself.

Indulge in gratitude
It is impossible to worry or be angry and grateful at the same time!
Practicing gratitude is one of the fastest and easiest ways to

* Shift your energy and mood from upset and stressed to happy and peaceful
* Manifesting more abundance and things to be grateful for!

Make use of your naturally occurring alpha brain state when you wake up and go to sleep at night.
End your day with positive thoughts. Even if you have had an awful day, you will find something to be grateful for – if only it is the fact that you are now snuggled up in your cozy bed! Take only high vibrations into your sleep time.

Positive thoughts promote better sleep, beautiful dreams and train your brain into attracting what you want more of. This is why our sleep programming and nightly brain training audios as so successful!

The moment you feel yourself waking up, don't jump out of bed or go switch on your cell phone. Take just a few minutes to think of something to look forward to. It can be as simple as your first cup of coffee or the warm shower. Then set an intention for the day. What are you going to make a point of appreciating today? Is it your spouse, the barista, the bus driver, or something about yourself? Which body part do you want to say thanks to? I like starting from the bottom up: with my feet. We all too often neglect them and take them for granted that I feel they deserve to be first on the thank you list. You can show your appreciation by spoiling them to a massage, your most comfortable pair of shoes or walking barefoot. Become aware of how they carry you through life every day and send them a mental thank you note.

Make a Body-Vision-Board

When communicating with your subconscious mind and the Universe you want to be as specific as possible. Formulate your goals in a clear and very precise way; the order "I want to lose weight" will never be as effective as "I want to lose 20 pounds by the 20th September 2015." When you are visualizing your new life in your new, healthy and slim body, make sure you do so in a "3D-Dolby-Surround-Sound" way; the more you incorporate emotions and feelings into your mind's film reel, the better. It's like adding the turbo effect to your manifestation powers. A very helpful way to make this process easier and more visible for yourself is to create your very own Body Vision Board

You need
- A large piece of poster board
- Some photographs of you looking happy (face only)
- Cut outs from magazines and brochures of role model bodies you like the look of and any other images, which represent your goals (apart from weight loss; like health, energy, happiness, love, success and abundance)

Now chose your favorite images and stick these onto the poster board. Make sure you replace your role model's faces for images of yourself. Don't worry about them looking strange or disproportional – the main objective is to have a clear vision of yourself with your desired body shape all on one page.

Take your time creating this board; make it look special! And when you are done, hang it somewhere you will see it often (i.e. in the office or bathroom) Every time you look at your body board repeat some of your affirmations and create a happy, grateful feeling inside of yourself. Imagine what you feel like when you have achieved your goals and don't stop your manifestation session until you are grinning from ear to ear!

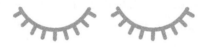

10 How your Best Friends can be your Worst Enemies in Weight Loss

H ave you ever experienced the following: You have just started out on your new weight loss regime, are highly motivated and are certain it's going to work this time. Actually you have already stuck to it longer than you thought you could! You are doing well, have lost some weight and people are noticing how good you look.

And then suddenly you are invited out for dinner, given a box of chocolates, or sent a gift voucher for an ice cream parlor – all by your closest friends! Or even worse: you accompany your usual crowd to your favorite diner and are managing to hold up strong; are happily chomping away on your salad, when your dear friends start their persuasion campaign: "Oh, come on! Don't be such a spoil sport... have some dessert...you must be hungry after just eating that salad... you're getting all skinny and crabby, you look older/sick...I liked you better when you were a little rounder...you've got to have some pleasure in life... you're no fun to be with any more ever since you're on this diet..." And all of a sudden you feel bad about not joining in, worried about disappointing them and before you know it, you put your newly gained willpower aside and order dessert. Does any of that sound familiar?

The crab effect in weight loss

Recent studies revealed that women seem to be masters at applying the crab technique, when their female friends start out on a weight loss regime.

New research by Vouchercloud.com has revealed that the average Briton loses two friends for every stone of weight lost during a diet? Why? Jealousy!

The money saving site polled 2,547 UK residents, all of whom were aged 18 or over and had been on a diet over the last 18 months which resulted in a weight loss of one stone or more. When asked about the negative effects they had experienced as a result of losing weight, 81% revealed they had lost friends during the course of their weight loss journey.

As soon as a friend starts shedding the extra fat, we try to sabotage their efforts in weight loss. You see, nobody wants to be the fattest in a group of friends. When one of our fellow friends starts shedding the extra pounds, and gets a grip on their weight (and life!), we feel left out. It makes us feel uncomfortable because it feels like someone close to us has left our circle of comfort zone. And we automatically try and pull them back into our circle.

But not only our female friends apply this technique, so do our spouses. In fact, in one survey, 24,000 overweight women reported that weight loss created problems in their relationships that regaining the weight would have resolved.

What is the crab mentality?

Take a bucket full of crabs. If one crab attempts to escape from the bucket of live crabs, the other crabs will pull it back down, rather than allowing it to get free. Often, the crabs will wait until the courageous one has nearly escaped before pulling it back into the bucket. It's an odd phenomenon and relates to us humans. Why do we more often pull each other down, instead of supporting each other's growth?

When a person changes, it automatically has us look at our selves. And the mirror goes up really without anyone doing anything. People question their path, what they are doing and if what they think is "right" still holds true. So if you are changing (and funnily enough it's often our outside world who notices these changes before we do), your environment has to a) check in with themselves and b) is confronted with the possibility of you moving on, i.e. leaving them. This especially holds true with weight loss, as this is a very <u>visible</u> change. You can't keep this shift secret for very long (as opposed to a more internal growth process) and people will automatically start commenting on your change.

Additionally people will usually fiercely defend their current beliefs for 3 reasons:

1. They don't have enough information
2. They feel threatened
3. They are scared because if their beliefs don't hold true any more, they have to change too. And change is scary, remember? It entails going into the unknown and that can feel terrifying.

Roy's story of being a vegetarian

As a practicing holistic medical doctor way back in 1980 I became a devoted vegetarian. I grew up in a meat-loving family in which the pecking order was revealed by the size of the steak you would get on your plate. My father got always the biggest portion of animal protein then came my oldest brother and after that: me. We were a family of 10, as my father was a devout catholic and the pope wanted big families and no birth control. After reading several studies revealing how consuming red meat and animal protein could cause serious chronic illnesses and seeing many patients recover after going meat-less, I decided to become a vegetarian. At that time it was still a rarity. For my family it was total shock, and for 2 years at every occasion possible I would be mocked and offered all kinds of meat dishes that used to be my favorites. When I also lost weight and could show off a six-pack beach body, the efforts to tempt me with all kinds of foods and desserts increased 4 fold. My mother was really worried because I was so skinny and asked me many times if I was OK and that she was sad that I was no longer her old chubby boy. It was not hard for me to say no to temptation as my medical experience never left any space for doubt. So I became good at bringing my own favorite dishes to eat or started to prepare a meal instead of getting only potatoes with an onion sauce or a plate full of overcooked veggies as a meal. My dislike for cooked dead and tasteless meals, high in salt and spices grew and even the most intrinsic spices could not bring them back to a level that my palate would recognize as edible. I had become so used to fresh, vital food that I craved it. After 3 years everyone finally accepted that my fad was not going away and I noticed that now my hosts would really do their best to make a wholesome vegetarian meal for me. This is when I knew that finally they had come full circle and it was fun to see that they would also regularly serve a vegetarian dish for the whole family. My advice to you: Stick to your nutritional regimen and become good at saying no to undesired offerings of temptations.

Joy's snippet

My story of opting for a vegetarian lifestyle is similar. I went off meat when I was 14, was also confronted with disapproval and concern by my family, who were worried that their daughter wasn't getting enough nutrients and protein. I am blessed to have a tolerant family; my parents quickly shifted their opinion and after a while even went out of their way to accommodate my eating habits. I was always interested in trying out different nutritional approaches and there is not much I didn't try. After seeing me test the umpteenth variation of what to eat and what not, I guess I was stamped off as slightly crazy and my surrounding merely raised an eyebrow upon hearing about my latest fad. My take is: do your research and test what feels right for you. Every body is different. Some people thrive on a vegetarian or even vegan diet; others do better if their diet contains some organic meat. Once you are truly listening to your body again, you will get almost instant feedback from it and quickly learn what is best for you. It's not rocket science: If you feel tired, sick or "off" after your meals, you are doing something wrong. Check out what this something is; leave out what you suspect is causing you discomfort and replace it with another wholesome, natural food. You will soon discover what "diet" gives you energy, promotes well being and keeps you at a healthy weight.

You are the reflection of the 5 people closest to you

Tune in to what frequency those 5 peeps are vibrating at and you'll get a good indicator of where you're at {or where you were}. Are all your friends overweight? What issues, areas in life are they struggling with? What similarities do your problems have? It can give you some valuable insights answering these questions for yourself.

As we start to grow, our frequencies change. We simply vibrate differently. And if we try to cover up that "being different" with a mask of "sameness," pretending to be like our peer group because we are terrified of getting expelled… it usually backfires. If you pretend to be someone you are not, you are lacking integrity. To yourself and others. Not being authentic does not pay off! We go against ourselves, playing a role that doesn't resonate with who we truly are. Keeping up appearances burns up a lot of energy and creates stress in our systems. At best we feel tired, worst case we get sick. And in most cases we get found out anyway. People sense more than they know or can consciously explain. And if you are sending out incongruent messages/vibrations, they will start feeling uneasy about and with you.

If the people closest to you represent who you were a while back, it may be time to lovingly detach and change the Rolodex. Maybe they will change with you but don't count on it. Now, don't get us wrong: we are NOT suggesting you drop all your overweight friends! But we do want you to be aware of the crab phenomenon and pay attention if it is affecting your efforts in weight loss.

Protect your energy and enthusiasm

You might want to rethink who you share your new ideas, thoughts, and goals with. Not everybody is ready to understand the concept of managing your weight with the power of your mind. And it doesn't really matter if they don't; the only person, who truly matters in this process, is: YOU! You can lose weight in your sleep. You are redefining what is possible. You are utilizing the power of your mind. You are reconnecting to your natural skinny and healthy self. You are a success story. Period.

Some people are great to talk to as soon as you have an inspiration, they are valuable sounding boards, encouraging and uplifting. Others are better informed once you are successful and have achieved your desired weight.

And remember: Nobody can hold you back or have any influence in your life if you do not (in some way or other) give permission to do so. They can only have the impact you are allowing them to have.

The ones that matter will understand and the ones that don't, don't matter.

Everybody has their own time frame and way of doing things, also when it comes to weight loss. Some people are ready to tackle their weight issues, others are not – make sure you don't turn into a walking weight loss preacher, forgetting your role as a friend. Lead the way by being a shining example of courage, wisdom, and love. Inspire your friends by being a role model of health and vitality and be there to support them when they are ready.

Mary's story

Mary, a 42-year-old woman, had been kind of round ever since she was a teenager. When she started becoming conscious of herself, she did not like what she saw in the mirror. She did not believe she was attractive and saw herself as inferior to the cool girls in school. To add to the insult, her family was not very rich and she could not wear the cool outfits her peers had. She became more and more depressed and started to copy her mother's behavior. Her mother was not feeling happy because she was working day and night to keep everything going, was frustrated that her work was not being seen and she was taken for granted. She was always complaining and could make quite some scenes about little things. The marriage was not one of great romance or an example of intimacy or closeness. Her father was a hard working employee of a phone company, was always tired when he came home and his biggest reward was TV and beer. So her mother literally ate her frustrations away and had a knack for ice cream and muffins. She would eat bran-muffins because those were healthy and were good for bowel movements. She was increasing in size every year and ballooned into the obesity numbers.

Mary also started to eat her frustrations away and developed this love hate relationship with chips and fried foods. She would binge on chips and donuts and then starve herself for a week and at the first sign of trouble go back to the fried foods. She came to see us at an obese weight of 170 pounds at 5.5' height.

She was married with someone she met in college and her marriage was going in the same direction as her mom's, with an exception: she had no children.

We started working on her addiction to chips and fried foods, breaking the emotional patterns she had suffered from for so long. After 2 sessions she was ready for a virtual gastric band (see chapter 6) and after that she was losing weight steadily and graciously, around 4-6 pounds every month. She enjoyed the process! In one of our follow up sessions she was telling us how strange the reactions of her female colleagues and her mom were to her. Most of her colleagues were overweight.

All the 9 over-sized colleagues were worried about her that she was losing weight too fast and that she might be sick. They were asking her out for dinner much more frequently than ever before and always wanted to go to the 'all you can eat' restaurants specializing in fried foods. They would even bring in some of her former favorite dishes for her, urging her to indulge in "some of the good stuff." Mary however was so well prepared on a subconscious level to follow the simple guidelines of naturally thin people; she would stop eating as soon as she felt satisfied and even if others would move heaven and earth, try to make her feel guilty… she would not eat more. She said she was surprised at how steadfast she was, how easy it was to say no and not feel guilty. She said: "My biggest victory is that I can leave food on my plate and actually feel happy doing so. Every time I leave food on my plate it feels like a total victory, I enjoy that so much; I can finally say no to overeating. The second victory is that I can stare chips in the face without feeling any temptation or craving whatsoever. They do not call my name any more and I know that the relationship we once had is over!"

We are so proud of her because she is a great example that when you get the subconscious mind to work with you, there is no need for willpower and struggle any more! We love what we do because it is rewarding to hear stories like Mary's.

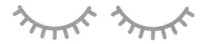

11

Drink Water
and Lose Weight

The placebo effect: power of expectation and belief

I n our program, your mind is trained to believe that drinking water is THE tool to lose weight. It is not about what you consciously think is true or false. The body follows what you subconsciously believe to be true or what you expect to happen. In science this is called the placebo effect. If you give a person a medicine that is supposed to calm them down and tell them it will stimulate them to have lots of energy (the opposite effect), depending on the charisma and congruency of the person giving the medicine, the suggested effect can be achieved in over 90% of the test-persons. They will feel energized and stimulated instead of sedated and without energy.

In other words:

What you believe is more powerful than the chemical effect of the given potion! This has created a new science: mind-body-healing. Actually it is very old and has been done by shamans and healers all over the world for centuries. In many cases the power of these healers can be stronger than the best medicine!

New medicines are always tested against placebo effect. Many pharmaceutical medicines do not pass this test, as the placebo effect is much stronger than the chemicals tested. In other words if you believe something is good for you or if you believe it is bad for you: in both cases your belief will shape the effects of the chemical or medicine. And sometimes people have given up hope and they stop believing.

Your mind creates your reality. Start with an open mind!

In hypnosis this is taken to another level and can be so powerful that the mind can anesthetize the body completely to the point that surgery can be done without painkillers. Hypnosis makes you relax to a state you can compare with meditation and you are not filtering the information from what you have learned. Instead you have an open mind to consider everything as a possibility and let go what you discover is no longer at your best interest. When hypnosis is done properly, you can go back to any event in your history and look at it with fresh eyes and not filter it by your past conditioning. This means that you can change the meaning of that event and so change your personal past. This effect can have a great healing effect of traumatic experiences.

The broken vase syndrome

Let us for a moment assume your father yelled at you when you broke a vase in the living room as a child. You were so shocked and felt so bad because you saw the disappointment in your father's vase that you draw some conclusions that then became beliefs. Your first conclusion was that your father is right: you are clumsy and never pay attention. The second one is that you believe your father does not love you any more and thirdly, you have to proof that you are unworthy of his love.

Imagine that this happens when you are 5 years old; can this have a deep effect on your life? Can this result in you having negative self talk every time something goes wrong and you say to yourself: "Here I go again, I can't do anything right, I am clumsy!" Also you are likely to develop lower self-esteem and will always try to proof that you are worthy of love. You always tend to believe that people don't love you because you are not worthy of their love. So you go out of your way to try to please people and always feel inferior.

And this is just 1 broken vase. Imagine a series of events shaping your destiny, especially in the vulnerable age up to seven, when you cannot filter the reality properly but react from your emotional experience. You create beliefs around your emotions to explain to yourself what they mean. With hypnosis we can go back to that incident and you can now look at what happened with fresh eyes, equipped with more life experience (you understand why your father was mad and what made him blurt out what he did and understand that he didn't really mean what he was saying) and give that incident a complete new meaning. By doing that you immediately change how you feel, what you believe about yourself and form a new self-image.

Hypnosis is one of the most powerful techniques to change your personal history. You can't change what happened but you can change the meaning you gave to an incident. Thus you change how you feel in the now about certain issues in your life and so create a new experience of reality that is no longer based on your old beliefs!

That is very powerful and very healing! And it also explains why we love our brain training programs. They are based on the same principles: changing the way we feel by eliminating old patterns that influence us!

Why is drinking water so important?

As we mentioned several times, over the course of our lifetime most of us have moved away from our natural instincts. In our genetic programming we are predestined to drink water when we are thirsty. There is no genetic programming to drink soft drinks or even freshly squeezed orange juice.

A side step to the trend of drinking fresh juices and smoothies

These fruit, veggie and protein bombs have become increasingly popular and you can get them almost everywhere. As healthy and nutritious these might be, it is essential to see them as what they really are: a meal replacement! They are not designed to be the replacement of water or serve as a drink! We have seen many health conscious clients fall for this trap and so consume many more calories and far too much sugar and acid than is good for them just from drinking their daily smoothies and juices additionally to their regular diet.

When we break the genetic code of our inborn thirst mechanism, we also disrupt the feedback mechanism in the body that regulates our thirst center. So when we are thirsty and we give the body a drink that is not water (or unsweetened herbal tea), the body gets confused and deregulated. Thus we are creating a conditioning to look for a "tasty" drink or something to eat, when our body actually needs hydrating with plain water.

Hunger and thirst

If you have ever eaten everything in sight, yet didn't feel satisfied afterwards, you might have experienced receiving mixed brain signals. The hypothalamus controls both hunger and thirst, so it sends the same signal whether you are hungry or thirsty. To understand which signal your brain is sending, you must learn to understand your body better. Pay close attention to that feeling you have inside when you think you are hungry. It might be that empty feeling in your stomach only needs some water for satiety.

By drinking sugared drinks or even so called healthy drinks we are loading the body with calories and sugars it does not need and which will turn into fat. Research has shown that to cleanse the body of excess toxins nothing beats water! By starting to drink more water we are helping our body to detox and that will give us more energy!

The power of the mind unleashed once more

In the mental programming/brain training we have created, we stimulate the drinking of water as an effective way to curb hunger and stimulate the burning of fat by increasing the metabolism.

Over the years of your lifetime you have stored toxins in your body. These are stored in the organs, the ligaments, and the fat tissue. As you are now starting to burn fat in an accelerated speed, you dislodge the toxins from the fat tissues and they circulate in the blood and lymph. By drinking water we flush them out of the body and because of that your vitality will increase and you will feel better. This also translates in feeling less hungry and feeling more energy. When you add to the normal effects of water, your mind power of believing that water can help you burn more energy and thus burn more of the fat cells, we get a double effect. The mind just needs something to hold on to. It is much easier to tell someone that the pill they get will help them heal than to tell them they can heal themselves. So if you believe that water will help you burn fat, you will experience water as a fat burning solution, just like the placebo effect!

Water is the best fat burning elixir

So how is this done? In the programming we create you will link water to fat burning! By creating a strong neuro-chemical reaction in your brains each time you drink water you can increase the metabolic rate and this will result in turning the body into an efficient fat burning machine. Because of this new empowering belief, which is programmed in your nervous system, water becomes your best friend. Every time you drink water, you are decreasing your feelings of hunger and increasing your fat burning capacity. An added effect is that the more you burn fat, the less hungry you become because your blood sugar level becomes more stable. As an effective fat burner you will have less emotional swings because it is often low blood sugar that makes you more emotionally vulnerable. Your body is stimulated to burn fat as the best way to get energy. When that happens you feel less hungry and you don't depend on sugar to feel good!

A win-win situation: walk more, burn more!

Drinking water has so many benefits that it should be your number one drink every day and you will notice you will drink at least 10 full glasses of water every day. We recommend you drink 3 liters of water; the best way to do that is to have 3 1-liter bottles ready in the morning. We recommend you drink the first liter before 10.00 am. The next liter of water you drink before 14.00 and then the rest in the afternoon. Yes, you are right: you will go to the bathroom more often, but the added benefit of that is that you get to walk more. And that also burns more calories; see it as a positive thing! You can put some fresh lemon juice in your water if you like. You can drink it at room temperature, cold or warm, whatever you please.

What kind of water?

Mineral water is the best, but any water is better than diet drinks, soft drinks, juices, alcohol, or coffee. So do not get too hung up about what water to drink, just drink water instead of all other drinks, and drink a minimum of 3 liters per day. Within 2 weeks you will notice 4 things:

4. You will have more energy and feel more vital
5. You will start losing weight faster!
6. Your skin will look fresher and be more hydrated
7. Your digestive system will work better, you will eliminate more effortlessly

For coffee drinkers

If you drink coffee, drink an extra glass of water after your cup of coffee, because coffee dehydrates your body. If you drink alcohol it is the same. If you want to drink something warm, just drink warm water with lemon or unsweetened (preferably herbal) tea. There are also some really good herbal teas out there that have added benefits. One of our favorites is holy basil tea (also called Tulsi tea) Have fun trying out new tastes! Also tasty is adding some fresh ginger to hot water – a great stimulant and booster for your immune system.

Morning water with lemon

By drinking lemon water first thing in the morning, you will not only be able to give your digestive system a little kick start, but you will also benefit from a whole list of health related bonuses. Listed below are the amazing benefits that come along with drinking just one cup of hot lemon water each morning. It's as simple as boiling a pot of water, and adding a slice of lemon!

Boost your immune system

Loading up on vitamin C is a great way to fight against colds during peak flu seasons, and lemons are loaded with just that! In addition, lemons are very high in potassium, which is known for stimulating nerve and brain function, as well as controlling blood pressure. Vitamin C is also an antioxidant that protects your blood vessels against plaque.

Balance pH

Lemon has to be one of the most alkaline foods out there, and by drinking lemon water daily; you can reduce the overall acidity inside of your body. Acidity can cause wear and tear of joints and fatigue. It is good to know that the citric acid found in the lemon once metabolized will not create acidity in the body. In addition, studies have shown that people who maintain a more alkaline diet tend to shed more pounds far quicker than those who don't.

Reduce hunger cravings

Lemons rate quite high in pectin fiber, which helps fight hunger cravings. Now you have the effect of water and lemon combined to reduce you hunger!

Digestion

Lemon juice helps flush out all of those unwanted, indigestible materials. In fact, lemon water encourages the liver to produce bile which is an acid required for digestion. Lemon can help in the reduction of both constipation and heartburn.

Natural diuretic: flush out toxins

Warm lemon water in the morning will increase urination, resulting in flushing more toxins out!

Clear skin

The vitamin C in lemons can help decrease both blemishes and wrinkles. Lemon water literally eliminates harmful toxins from the blood, allowing your skin to remain crystal clear. In addition, to help reduce the appearance of scars, you can apply lemon directly on the area of concern.

Fresh breath

Lemon water can relieve gingivitis, tooth pain, and even keep your breath nice and fresh. Since hot lemon water is quite refreshing, why not skip that morning coffee and opt for a cup of hot lemon water to wake you up and keep your breath fresh.

Relieve respiratory problems

Simply put, hot lemon water can help heal chest infections, coughs, and has even shown success with patients of allergies and asthma.

Keeping you ZEN

When your body has encountered stress, Vitamin C is one of the first things to deplete. Drink a cup of lemon water daily, and you will be chocked full of Vitamin C.

Helping you kick the coffee habit

Trying to get away from drinking obscene amounts coffee for more reasons than one? After a glass of hot lemon water, your morning coffee cravings will slowly disappear. It's hard to explain, but it works!

Make this a new habit to kick start your day

Make drinking lemon water a regular habit, go ahead and swap out the daily cup of java for a nice hot cup of lemon water. You will see and feel the power of the lemons in little to no time.

Joy's extra tip:

Try spicing your lemon water (and your metabolism!) up by adding a sprinkle of Cayenne pepper. I am also a big fan of doTERRA's "Slim and Sassy" oil blend. One of the great things about these oils is that you can take them internally as well as using them externally. I add just one drop of "Slim and Sassy" to my glass (!) water bottle and adore the refreshing taste. This blend was created to boost your metabolism and help you turn into a fat burning machine. If you are interested in getting a little bottle of yummy-ness, please go here: https://www.mydoterra.com/joymartina/

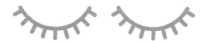

12

Busting the Myths on Eating and Metabolism

We were all brought up with certain rules and myths and many of these are passed on from generation to generation. You see this effect also with bodybuilders, who ingest ridiculous amounts of protein and pills to grow big muscles. Most of this is based on myths rather than research or scientific proof.

In this chapter, we are going to look at some of the myths that keep you a prisoner in a fat body.

Myth #1 Breakfast is the most important meal of the day!

This is a big one. Breakfast is the most important meal of the day…right?

This myth was originally created to sell eggs and bacon as THE American breakfast and has, in combination with cheap subsidized junk food, made America the world champion nation in obesity.

Our culture has bought into the myth, stating that if we don't eat a good breakfast we will suffer the following consequences:

1. Our metabolism slows down
2. We'll get intense cravings and lose energy
3. It will be harder to lose weight and burn fat

Joy and I were both brought up in that philosophy and I remember gobbling down on all the oatmeal in the morning and getting as much in as possible! The mandatory glass of orange juice or milk for vitamin C or calcium was an added supplement to our breakfast! I would feel drugged when walking to school and by 10.00 a.m. I would be ravenously hungry again and thank God I had a sandwich or snack to make that right!

Breakfast became an even bigger feast in our family when we got chickens and we had eggs with bacon every morning that was extra yummy! That part actually helped with the hunger feelings around 10.00 a.m.; they moved to 11.00 a.m.

Now, I'll be the first one to admit that for a very long time I was a huge advocate of eating breakfast as a healthy way to start your day and get your metabolism moving. Even as a medical doctor I did not know better and I was preaching the breakfast religion.

But over the last 15 years, published scientific researches, using real world people (instead of mice, rats and monkeys), are now showing a totally different picture. It is sad that the medical community and dieticians have still not caught up on this and are still preaching the old myth!

Over 3 years ago I started changing my approach to eating breakfast for health reasons and fat loss ... often skipping it all together. Since I started with this, it became easier for me to stay lean and it's MUCH easier to adhere to my Sleep Your Fat Away approach of listening to my body.

Joy: My family was definitely part of the breakfast gang; as kids we had to eat breakfast – hungry or not. On weekends my mum would even make the extra effort of cooking us waffles or other delicious things. And we sure loved our Sunday brunches!

With time I got used to morning routine and dutifully ate my bowl of cereal every day. Yet not only was I already tired after breakfast but ravenous come snack time at school. So once I became a slightly rebellious teenager, I switched to eating a piece fruit for breakfast, which I found to be far more energy giving than toast or cereal. When I started studying the low sugar approach on life, I ditched the fruit for green tea and/or a green smoothie for breakfast and found this to be even better.

Today I get up early (around 5.30), work out and stick to green tea until around 9 a.m. and find that this enhances my morning performance and eradicates mid morning sugar low. Our kids have adopted this routine and drink their smoothies before they head off for school. I like the idea that their smoothie contains their portions of greens, vitamins, and protein for the day and we have found this also greatly improves their morning mood. And to be honest: I'll do a lot to be saved from grumpy kids in the morning!

The 3 lies we have been told about breakfast

LIE #1: Breakfast Increases Your Metabolism

The whole idea that by not eating a big breakfast you will somehow slow down your metabolism is a big hype of false B.S. (B.S. stands for belief systems)

What really will change your life is following the Sleep Your Fat Away program and recognizing three basic truths:

A. The actual amount of calories you're taking in on a daily basis (Quantity)
B. The composition of those calories (Quality)
C. The amount of energy you burn every day

As long as you're making healthy choices regarding what you put in your mouth and keeping your body in a calorie deficit, it really doesn't matter much WHEN you eat those calories.

Proof: In a recent paper published in the American Journal of Clinical Nutrition, researchers delved into dozens of studies to uncover the relationship between eating breakfast and losing body weight.

Conclusion: The researchers concluded that breakfast being the most important meal of the day is merely a shared belief (B.S.). In other words, there is ZERO long-term research indicating or proving that eating breakfast leads to lower body fat or increased metabolism.

LIE #2: Eating a Good Breakfast Helps Control Your Hunger

As I already told you before, eating a big oatmeal breakfast made me hungrier than not eating anything or eating some protein in the morning. The ritual of eating breakfast first thing in the morning to increase energy levels and help you stave of cravings is the exact opposite of what happens in reality. The reason (and this completely resonates with our stories) is that a typical breakfast will spike insulin levels and send your blood sugar peaking sky high! This does two detrimental things to your health and waistline: the sugar drop that follows the high will cause a hunger binge, putting your body in a fat storing mode. Secondly, over time you will develop what is called insulin sensitivity decrease, which means that your body becomes less sensitive to the insulin, and all the sugar goes straight into fat storage. This is one of the biggest reasons for today's worldwide obesity, thanks to our fast and junk food society. Eating a big breakfast eventually will _decrease_ your sensitivity to insulin and _increase_ your appetite.

LIE #3: Breakfast Helps You with Weight loss

There are tons of studies and claims that eating a big, well-balanced breakfast helps promote weight loss. But in reality there are NO long-term studies that show a direct correlation between eating a healthy breakfast and weight loss. Maintaining a calorie deficit, making wise food choices and increasing your level of activity are all that really matters when it comes to staying healthy and losing fat.

The 3 Truths

Truth #1

What we will show later is that skipping breakfast will force your body to burn all the sugars in your reserve and then start to burn fast. The longer the time between your last meal (the day before) and your first next meal (breaking the fast), the more you will turn your body into a fat burner. The key is to stay away from carbs for as long as possible.

Truth #2

The second truth is that a big breakfast is a tremendous toll on your metabolic system; it decreases your productivity and slows you down. Think of the times when you had a big breakfast (most of us do this on vacation when we are staying at a hotel that serves an enticing breakfast buffet or other all you can eat options). How did you feel afterwards? Rearing to go, ready for some exercise? Or are you more tired and ready to hit the beach lounger? Many people have been forced to eat breakfast even when they were not hungry in the morning.

Truth #3

Skipping or postponing breakfast for as long as you can, will allow you to reverse your strategy so you will improve your insulin sensitivity and increase your fat burning. Your main caloric intake then is dinner—as long as you follow the rules of eating only when hungry and to stop eating when fulfilled!

Yes, you can still have a light breakfast if you want—this is not an intermittent fasting approach, just avoid carbohydrates if you want to speed up weight loss— if you can until dinnertime!

This system is called Early Morning Depletion, which will keep your body in fat-burning mode all day long.

Over time we noticed that we are seldom hungry early in the morning. We start feeling a little hungry around 10.00-11.00 am and really hungry around 12.00 to 1.00 pm. Remember the first rule of the naturally thin person is to only eat when hungry. So if you are not hungry, do not eat. And stop eating as soon as you feel satisfied. Stuffing yourself with a big breakfast is a big No-No!

What is a good breakfast?

Here you will find that the opinions are divided. What we can tell you is that it is not a good idea to combine protein with carbs. So no eggs with bread, grits and potatoes.

Most people feel much better with a light breakfast. This can be oatmeal (without sugar) mixed with some blueberries and strawberries, add some Chia seeds and Flax seeds for extra fiber. Some people like just fruits in the morning; we advise you to not mix too many fruits. Keep berries with berries maybe add some melons or a banana. And watch out for fruits that contain a lot of sugar like bananas.

Do not drink a large glass of orange juice in the morning on a regular basis. These are wasted calories, which go straight to your waist; unsweetened green tea or red tea (rooibos) is better. Another alternative is cereal (natural organic non processed cereals) with almond milk or rice milk and some berries. Avoid eating lots of bread, pancakes or processed foods in the morning. Green smoothies are a great alternative, which can be a mixture of super foods like broccoli, chlorella, kale, celery, and some natural protein. Try adding some coconut milk or water, lemon juice and half a banana! We are lovers of healthy smoothies and often replace breakfast and lunch with smoothies filled with healthy seeds, probiotics and greens or berries.

Two of our favorite "detox and slim" smoothies to kick start your day

Green Ginger
    1 cucumber
    1 celery stalk
    2 green apples
    2 handfuls of spinach
    ½ lemon, juiced

2 inches of fresh ginger root

1 cup of coconut water

You can also add some spirulina, wheat grass powder or chlorella. A piece of broccoli is also good! We love to add some flax seeds or psyllium husks!

Juice all the ingredients together and sip slowly!

Chia-Acai-Berry

3 cups strawberries

4 cups seedless grapes

2 tbsp acai powder

3 tbsp chia seeds

1 cup of coconut milk (optional)

We like adding some flax seeds or psyllium husks!

You can also add some vegan protein to make it even more filling!

Put all ingredients in a blender with ice cubes and enjoy!

Myth #2:"You need to eat every 3 hours to boost your metabolism."

We hear this myth very often. Especially when we talk about the benefits of intermittent fasting (IF).

A common form of IF is to postpone your breakfast till after noon (between 1.00 and 3.00 pm); some people go to the extreme and don't eat for one or two 24-hour periods per week, which helps you reduce your overall food intake by 14% to 28%. It is best to build this up over time; we like to do a detox day a week; this is a day where you only drink a lot of water and green smoothies, nothing else!

Like we said previously, eating healthy foods is the key to your health, but if you also want to burn fat you NEED to create a calorie deficit of some sort. We accomplish that by eating less without triggering the sabotage mechanisms in your body, by following the guidelines and having a virtual gastric band installed. This is like attacking the problem from 2 sides and you naturally reduce your intake. IF helps you to become more of a fat-burner by postponing your breakfast. Especially if you exercise in the morning, you will burn more sugar reserves in your body and force your body to burn fat. By not eating carbohydrates in the morning you will reach the same goals. That is why a green shake in the morning with no carbs is the best way to go, you can also add some coconut fat which will help you burn more belly fat.

Now, let us list some more myths we hear about fat loss, metabolism and IF, and send them running with a good kick in the rear... (Thanks to Brad Pilon, the author of "Eat Stop Eat" for his incredible research)

Myth #3:"Skipping meals reduces your metabolism."

This idea is made very popular by the food industry, but that's probably because they want you to believe that you NEED to eat every 3 hours or so to boost their sales of snacking foods.

In reality, many studies prove that your food intake has little to do with your metabolism, at least short term:

In one study, researchers found that when they made people fast for 3 days, their metabolic rate did not change. This is 72 hours without food!

In another study by a different group of researchers, people who fasted every other day for a period of 22 days also saw no decrease in their resting metabolic rate.

In still more studies, there was no change in the metabolic rate of people who skipped breakfast, or people who ate two meals a day compared to seven meals per day.

The bottom line is that the frequency of food intake has very little to do with your metabolism. In fact, your metabolism is much more closely tied to your body weight.

Myth #4: "Overweight people have a 'slow' metabolism"

This popular idea closely tied to Myth 2. In fact, if your weight goes up or down, so does your metabolism.

Yes, this means that the more fat your carry around, the higher your metabolism generally is—which means that you burn more fat when at rest.

Myth #5:"Exercising and fasting is exhausting or dangerous"

Note: If you suffer from some type of blood sugar issue (hypoglycemia, diabetes, etc.), this can be the case. Please check with your doctor before embarking on any weight loss and/or exercise regime!

But for healthy individuals, this is simply NOT true at all.

Already in 1987, researchers found that a three-day fast had no negative effects on how strongly your muscles can contract, your ability to do short-term high intensity exercises, or your ability to exercise at moderate intensity for a long duration.

This means that your body can tap into your multiple energy resources just fine even if you don't eat before exercise, and even when you didn't eat for 24 hours.

Myth #6: "You will lose your muscle mass if you skip meals or do IF (Intermittent Fasting)"

This statement is only true if you don't do some kind of resistance training. Think of hospital patients. After days of sitting in a bed and never using their muscles, their body naturally starts breaking down muscle tissue as energy because it basically concludes that these muscles are useless.

But if you do challenge your muscles with your favorite kind of exercise (weight lifting, yoga, body weight stuff, etc.), you won't lose any muscle mass while fasting or if you happen to skip a few meals.

Research on men and women on a very low calorie diet found that even with a 12 week long diet consisting of only 800 Calories and 80 grams of protein per day (which we don't recommend at all, but it was for the sake of research), the people in the study were able to maintain their muscle mass as long as they were exercising with weights three times per week.

In another study, men restricted their caloric intake by eating 1,000 Calories less per day than they normally ate for 16 weeks. They took part in a weight-training program three days a week and were able to maintain all of their muscle mass while losing over 20 pounds of body fat.

This doesn't mean that these very low calorie diets are healthy. The point is that calorie restriction does NOT lead to muscle loss if you challenge your muscles regularly.

Myth #7: "Intermittent fasting (IF) is unhealthy"

Again, the truth is the complete opposite.

IF shows many benefits like:

- Decreased body fat & body weight
- Maintenance of skeletal muscle mass
- Decreased blood glucose levels
- Decreased insulin levels & increased insulin sensitivity
- Increased fat oxidation
- Increased growth hormone levels
- Decreased food related stress

As you can see, IF is safe (except if you have a particular blood sugar condition) and very effective to help you reduce your overall calorie intake in a week.

The best thing: it will NOT slow your metabolism, burn your muscles (as long as you do resistance training rather than long cardio) or prevent you from exercising.

So if you think it would be a good addition to your fat loss routine, make sure you read the best resource on the subject: "Eat Stop Eat" by Brad Pilon. It's The Bible of Intermittent Fasting.

Let's look at one more issue:

Can eating too few calories stall your metabolism?

If you're like most people who want to **lose weight**, you want to lose it *fast*. So you may be tempted to make drastic changes in your diet to dramatically reduce the number of **calories** you consume. But what is common knowledge by now is that eating too few calories for a prolonged period can actually backfire and sabotage your weight-loss efforts.

There are two mechanisms at work that is important to understand. It is the difference between fasting and starvation. Why can monks be on a prolonged very low calorie diet and stay healthy? Because they are not starving, they honoring their foods, meditating (being in the alpha or theta brainwave state) a lot and are generally filled with gratitude. They have trained themselves to deal with their emotional issues and overcome inner sabotage. If you would eat the same meals without honoring the mental/mindful approach, you would feel hungry and go into the 3 D-triggers of Diet-Deprivation and Discipline.

Calories and your health

The most effective way to lose weight is to consume fewer calories than you expend, creating a calorie deficit. But if your calorie intake dips too low, your body could go into starvation (deprivation) mode. Your body will start to lower it's metabolism because it thinks it is not going to get enough food. That is why you will hit a plateau, the point where your body is kind of at a standstill.

When your body goes into deprivation mode, your metabolism slows to a crawl, burning calories as slowly as possible to conserve its energy stores. This is why people who cut down on their calories too much reach a plateau and stop losing weight. If this happens, you probably will become frustrated that your efforts are not paying off. This can then lead you to overeat or binge and ultimately gain weight. You just throw in the towel… Do you recognize this? It happens to over 66% of all people going on a diet!

In addition to sabotaging your weight-loss efforts, eating too few calories for a prolonged time can also harm your health. When your body goes into starvation mode, you are at increased risk for the following:

- Abnormally low blood pressure and slow heart rate
- Heart rhythm abnormalities
- Electrolyte imbalances, especially potassium deficiency
- Gallstones
- Hair loss
- Brittle fingernails
- Loss of menstrual periods in women

- Soft hair growth over entire body
- Dizziness
- Trouble concentrating
- Anemia
- Swelling in your joints
- Brittle bones
- Depression

Coming to terms with calories

Calories are not your enemy! They are a vital part of a healthy and energetic life. This is why fad diets that force you to cut out too many calories leave you feeling lethargic, shaky, and ready to give up.

That is why the Sleep Your Fat Away program is totally different, instead of following a fad diet, you will develop new reasonable eating habits and start moving your body more step by step; this allows most of our clients to lose a pound or two every week—consistently.

There is plenty evidence that people who lose weight at this rate by making better nutritional choices, eating smaller portion sizes, and exercising also have the best chance of keeping it off.

Make a plan to adopt new healthful habits that you will be able to stick to indefinitely, and always allow yourself a little wiggle room for special occasions.

Conclusion: Caveman science

Our real karma is that we have to live with the fact that our bodies are still genetically the same as those of our Cavemen ancestors.

Diet programs that claim fat loss of an average of 10-20 lbs. in 34 weeks (haven't we all seen these types of diets advertised over and over again) fail to tell you that you'd have to drastically cut calories for as much as 12 weeks if you want to lose any significant amount of weight.

So not only will you need to dramatically cut calories, but your metabolism will crash making it almost impossible to lose belly fat. You will lose muscle mass and gain frustration! That is why many people still don't lose weight despite eating way below their required caloric needs.

We have seen thousands people do it over and over (the law of insanity) and I have done it myself. Let's follow Einstein's advice and change our thinking and habits…. and succeed!

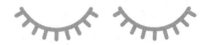

13

Exercise Can
Make You Fat!

E xercise is supposed to be good for weight loss and many people on the weight loss track will embark on all kinds of fitness regimen to lose weight. With every New Year come our possibly life changing resolutions. Among the top 10 of resolutions that people choose are to exercise more, lose weight, stop smoking and spend more time for self-reflection; by February most people are back to their normal routines and less than 15% will stick to their New Year's resolution.

55 Years of exercise

Roy: I have been in exercise and martial arts since the age of 6 and have trained thousands of people, worked with world champions and do know a thing or two about exercise. I have tried many different types of aerobics and fitness, weight training and stretching routines. What I am interested in now are the exercises that are most efficient in weight loss, prolong life (longevity) and increase endurance and muscle strength.

So let's look at several types of exercises and what effects they have. Let's start with the most famous one: aerobic exercise.

Aerobics

Lets start by busting this myth: Aerobics is good for weight loss.

Did you know that staying in the "fat-burning zone" promoted in aerobics can actually make you gain weight and fat? Fact is that you do burn calories but only when you exercise and there is no after-burn effect. Most people burn their sugar reserves first, so after exercising they may get hungry (sugar dip) and/or drink a sugar filled smoothie and the effect of 1 hour of aerobics is diminished.

Joe's story

25 years ago, I (Roy) was living in L.A. and every morning at 5.00 AM I would be in the gym with some martial arts students practicing special exercises to start our day. I was training them to become martial arts champions. We noticed that every morning we would see Joe at the gym. We spend around 2 hours in the gym working on martial arts training, boxing, flexibility etc. and Joe was always there too. One day I started a conversation with Joe and asked him about his routine. He would spend 3 and a half hours in the gym every morning (6 days a week), doing 2 aerobic classes and some weights, with a half hour break between the classes—effectively training almost 3 hours per day. Joe was obviously in great shape and I asked him why he was doing this. He said that it was the only way to keep his lifestyle. He loved eating a good meal, drink a few glasses of wine every evening, and in order not to put on weight he would work out from 5.00 am till 8.30 and then go to work. He said: "I hate dieting, so I found a way to eat what and as much as I want and still stay at the weight that I want. I am happy and I am super fit!" I don't think you will find many people like Joe, but they do exist. I know if I train twice a day I will lose weight, but it is not sustainable for a long period of time because of our schedule. There are options and more effective ways to stay on track than Joe's method.

So what about things like Crossfit?

In Crossfit people are pushed to their limits. Did you know that pushing too HARD for too LONG can backfire because you are unleashing a storm of age-accelerating inflammation within your body? Many believe that the Crossfit program that emphasizes high-volume, high-intensity workouts can lead to serious injuries. The culture of Crossfit pushes people beyond their limits and the high-intensity training can lead to a serious condition called rhabdomyolysis (rhabdo), in which muscle tissue breaks down and is carried by the bloodstream to the kidneys, which can't handle the load and shut down. Rhabdo is generally a very rare condition and Crossfit is the only sport, which has had to report several incidents of rhabdo. For many Crossfit can still be a good fit, but it is not recommendable for most people.

What about age? Can you be too old for exercise?

Millions wrongly believe they are too old, too out of shape or too injured to take advantage of exercise's powerful youth-enhancing ability to turn back the clock!

Let's begin with the worst workout

CARDIO or Aerobics exercises lead this category! This will certainly ruffle some feathers and bring down the holiness of the cardio industry, which has been promoted ever since Jane Fonda made it look sexy! The truth is that long boring cardio is officially the WORST workout you can do and of course you want to know why!

Why is cardio not good for you?

One of the reasons is that it is dead boring! Of course you can distract yourself with some upbeat music, watch CNN or a movie while sitting on an exercise bike or running on a treadmill for 45 minutes.

But much more important than the boring part is that cardio fails to produce good and permanent fat-loss RESULTS.

Are there health benefits? Sure. But you can get those same health benefits (and better ones) with much shorter, much more exciting and invigorating workouts. If you pay attention you will notice that even the commercials for cardio are changing. The industry is catching on to the science and understands that short and intense is better than long and boring!

More on that in a minute...

Joy's story

I was not an athletic kid. I didn't have athletic parents or other role models to introduce me to the sports side of life. Once my inborn desire for movement as a young child was replaced with the laziness of "teenagedom," I actually hated exercise. Sports classes at school made me feel inadequate and insecure. I felt everybody was better at sports than me and because I was growing increasingly unfit, I did not enjoy having to exert myself at all. I remember my sports teacher making me the laughing stock of the PE class one day when she called me "tomato-head." In our PE class we had to run up some small mountain and I was so out of breath that my face was bright red. So instead of going for it and start training, I chose to get out of exercise whenever I could. My saving grace was that I cycled to and from school every day, which at least gave me 1 hour of gentle movement in fresh air. Better than nothing but nowhere near enough to be able to take part in team sports or other really athletic activities. So my attitude towards sports and movement was that it was "painful and humiliating" and my belief was that I was simply no good at it. I decided to take on Winston Churchill's credo: "No sports."

I was 22 when I decided to start running. At that time "the" running guru Ulrich Strunz, was at large in Austria and Germany. I went to one of his lectures and was attracted to his theory that everyone can learn how to run and have fun while doing so. I decided to give it a go. I went from at first alternating running and walking for a few minutes at a time, to being able to take part in numerous organized charity runs. At last I had broken that limiting programming of "no sports" and for the first time thoroughly enjoyed moving! Actually I got so hooked to running that I had a hard time not being able to run for a day. I would get up at 5.30 in order to run before I woke my kids for school. Running was my salvation, my therapy, and "me time." I thought I had everything under control until one New Year's Day: I had been out for a run at 6 a.m., as usual, and was just arriving at my house, when my mother pulled up. I'll never forget how she looked at me, noticing my frozen eyelashes and eyebrows (it was -4° Fahrenheit that day) and said: "Have you ever asked yourself what you are running away from?" Bam! I was stunned. I took a critical look at myself and noticed how gaunt and skeleton-like I looked. I certainly did not look healthy! Today I know that I was draining my body with all this running. I was depleting my reservoirs and literally losing muscle.

That day I chose to stop this rather self destructive behavior, go within and find out what it was that I did not want to see. This triggered a big transformational process in my life and I was step by step able to tackle some big issues.

Today I realize how important the right kind of exercise and balance of all life's areas is. I no longer run for hours every day but focus on keeping a balance by doing weight training (kettle bells, with which I have love-hate relationship), short bursts of cardio (high intensity interval), daily stretching, yoga, and smart exercise routines. The result is that I look much better, have far more energy and am a happier, more peaceful and content person. My loved ones tell me I am much more pleasant to be with too!

Scientific research

But first, here's what research has to say about cardio:

Utter AC, et al. Influence of diet and/or exercise on body composition and cardio-respiratory fitness in obese women. Int J Sport Nutr. 1998 Sep;8(3): 213-22.

In this 3-month study, women did 45 minutes of cardio a day, 5 days a week, and lost no more weight than those who dieted alone! Seems like a royal waste of time me!

There are other researches proving that this one was not a fluke!

Redman et al. "Effect of calorie restriction with or without exercise on body composition and fat distribution." J Clin Endocrinol Metab. 2007 Jan 2.

In this study, subjects did 50 minutes of cardio, 5 days a week, and once again lost no more weight than those who dieted alone!

Well, maybe if we increase the duration to a full HOUR of cardio a day, SIX days a week, then cardio will actually produce substantial results? No again!

McTiernan et al. "Exercise Effect on Weight and Body Fat in Men and Women." Obesity 2007 June 15:1496-1512.

Over the course of this one year study, subjects performed aerobic exercise for 60 minutes a day, 6 whopping days a week (who even has TIME for that?) and lost only 3.5 pounds on average in an entire YEAR!

Ouch! That is lot of work! 312 hours of cardio is 13 days of cardio non-stop to lose no more than 3,5 pounds... this is the worst workout ever!

The good news

But we can heave a sigh of relief! There is a much better alternative: short, intense bouts of exercise achieve far better results.

In fact, a recent study published in the *European Journal of Applied Physiology* found that 15 minutes of an intense circuit-style resistance-training workout elevated the metabolism for a full THREE days! And that's only from 15 minutes! These are the kind of workouts you are looking for: something that is doable and has great long-term benefits.

More good news: longevity

Other studies have found similar results with interval style workouts as short as 4 minutes producing dramatically more fat loss than long, extended bouts of cardio. What I (Roy) discovered was even better news: when measured on the Heart Rate Variability (HRV), interval style workouts were much better in improving the HRV than any other type of exercise! Why is this important? Your HRV is an objective way to measure the intervals in between heartbeats. The more variation in between, the longer you will live. What this means is that your heart is better at adapting to changing circumstances. A child has a high HRV and it recovers quite quickly form exertion. The more you keep your heart rate constant in exercising, the worse the exercise. That is why running long distances like marathons are not good for your HRV compared to sprinting short distances; then recover and sprint again. So if you have an exercise bicycle, it is best to do a sprint with high load for 1 to 2 minutes 6 times, then have some recovery time in between. Don't sit cycling for one hour and cycle at a constant pace. Same goes for treadmills, ellipticals, climbers and other exercise devices.

Exercise intensity matters more than duration in keeping weight off

Every little bit counts. That's the message of a new study in the American Journal of Health Promotion, which showed that even a few minutes of brisk physical activity can add up to protect against obesity.

"What we learned is that for preventing weight gain, the intensity of the activity matters more than duration," study researcher Jessie X. Fan, a professor of family and consumer studies at the University of Utah, said in a statement. "This new understanding is important because fewer than 5 percent of American adults today achieve the recommended level of physical activity in a week according to the current physical activity guidelines. Knowing that even short bouts of 'brisk' activity can add up to a positive effect is an encouraging message for promoting better health."

Currently, U.S. adults are recommended to get 150 minutes of moderate to vigorous exercise a week. Using an accelerometer to gauge what this means, this could also be interpreted as getting to 2,020 accelerator counts per minute. In other words, this is the level of vigorous exercise you'd accomplish from walking at three miles per hour.

The study is based on data from the 2,202 women and 2,309 men ages 18 to 64 who were part of the National Health and Nutrition Examination Survey and who wore accelerometers from 2003 to 2006. Researchers found that the study participants fell into one of four categories of exercise intensity: higher-intensity long bouts, higher-intensity short bouts, lower-intensity long bouts, and lower-intensity short bouts.

They found that even the people who engaged in the higher-intensity short bouts experienced benefits to their body mass index. For instance, for women, spending an extra minute of high-intensity exertion each day was linked with a .07 decrease in body mass index.

Plus, for every additional minute of high-intensity exertion each day, obesity odds decreased by 5 percent for women and 2 percent for men.

Synergize exercise and nutrition

But here's the real secret...

NO workout will ever help you lose fat unless you get your nutrition in order. Unfortunately, nutrition is an area where most people really struggle, and sticking to a "diet" long term can be almost impossible.

But, have no fear... Sleep your fat away will break that cycle and get you going in a way that has not been done before.

Exercise should be apart of your daily routine but with the tips here you can do it in a short and intense way and get better benefits than doing long boring cardio.

Build up before you HIIT

Please note that it is crucial if you are out of shape (you have not done fitness for a while) to build up step by step (see later on the paragraph about walking). Sooner than later you then want to start increasing parts of your training to get the advantages of High Intensity Interval Training (HIIT)! This will be the best approach after getting the Sleep Your Fat Away program – so as soon as you have worked yourself up to be ready for HIIT (normally if you start at zero then this should be within 4 weeks).

How do you know if what you are doing is working?

You should know of the 3 metabolic signals that let you know if your efforts are working... or just a WASTE of time. In fact, when you follow these 3 signals, you can stimulate your metabolism to burn fat at an accelerated rate for up to 72 hours AFTER you workout. And new research shows that when you pay attention to these 3 signals, you can optimize your efforts to produce the fat-burning, muscle-toning results that you want, in as little as 6-15 minutes. This you can do at ANY age. Personally I love to exercise to the point of sweating and I seldom exercise under 20 minutes, but if I have no time or when travelling I can get the same results in 4 minutes top! The whole idea is to get what is called "the after burn effect"! The other thing is to take breaks when working and to do like 2 minutes in between a couple of times a day.

Metabolic Signal #1: Trigger the after-burn-effect...for days!

Here's the no.1 key to unleashing your metabolism's ability to burn fat and shape muscle: get out of breath. This is because of the anaerobic effect of intense interval workouts. That means doing exercise at the level of what is high intensity for you ensures that your heart and lungs are sufficiently activated. The fitter you are, the more intense the work out will be in order to get you breathless. You see, when you get out of breath, a metabolic alarm bell is triggered that releases catecholamines. Now, catecholamines are known as your "gas pedal" hormones. They instruct your body to break apart stored body fat and burn it for energy, pouring gas on to your metabolic fire.

A 2002 study in the European Journal of Applied Physiology shows that a special type of short, smart workout can get you breathless, elevating your metabolic rate by up to 21% in the 24-48 hours after you workout.

This equals DAYS of elevated fat burning, so make sure you get breathless more often!

Metabolic Signal #2: Unleash the burn-effect during exercise

Scientists used to think the burning sensation experienced during workouts was a sign of waste products (lactic acid) building up. Instead, research from the July 2009 British Journal of Sports Medicine shows this burning sensation is a metabolic signal that triggers simultaneous fat loss AND muscle growth. It does this by signaling your body to release HGH (Human Growth Hormone), your #1 youth-enhancing hormone. HGH is responsible for wrinkle-free skin, limitless energy, strong bones and an attractive body shape. Efficient workouts that last only minutes release a storm of this metabolic trigger, causing a surge in HGH and other anti-ageing hormones that help turn back the clock. So if you want to stay young, full of energy and attractive... pay attention to the burn!

Our fat burning mantra

So, when you feel it burn, you can in your mind say to yourself: I am burning fat, I am a fat burning machine and I am getting younger and younger and healthier and healthier. We called this our burn-mantra!

Metabolic Signal #3: Boost your mood and motivation

No doubt you've already experienced this signal when lifting something heavy. The straining, huffing, and puffing are all signs you're activating type II muscle fibers. And that's important because a May 2008 study by Hulmi et al. shows this triggers testosterone production, important both for men AND women. Testosterone helps women strengthen bones and prevent osteoporosis, while also providing a big lift to mood by relieving stress and anxiety. For men, testosterone boosts drive and motivation and builds nicely sculpted muscles and a powerful physique.

That's crucial because in men AND women testosterone plunges as we age. So make sure you leverage the heavy effect; you don't need ANY weights. Your own body weight works phenomenally well when using "intelligent" metabolic workouts (more below).

How do I start?

So if what everyone is doing is NOT burning fat and producing results... what IS? The answer is to get breathless, get the burn, and go heavy... ALL at the same time, all in the same workout, in the LEAST amount of time possible.

Here's an example body weight, short-burst exercise routine that you can try today to boost your metabolism and your fat loss results. We like doing this routine whenever we travel and there is no gym nearby or we don't have time to go.

Joy & Roy's travel work-out

    30 seconds of prisoner squats

    30 seconds of push-ups

    30 seconds of jumping jacks

    Repeat 3 to 4 times.

Over time, as you get fitter you can extend each exercise up to 1 minute! Later add burpees to it. The goal is to do each one for 1,5 minutes and then go to the next one.

You can find a short video showing this routine on our websites www. christallin.com and www.sleepyourfataway.com

This workout only takes SIX minutes and you'll burn way more fat than you will with those long, drawn out, boring cardio sessions.

Joy & Roy's 6 minute travel workout optimizes all 3 signals... Not in separate hour-long daily sessions that suck up all your playtime. And not in super-high intensity "infomercial" workouts that have you jumping around like a crazy person, putting you at severe risk for injuring your knees, shoulders or lower back.

Not only that, the powerful metabolic stimulus provided by these SMART movements unleashes a shock wave of fat burning and muscle-shaping that lasts for 2-3 days AFTER the workout.

I've seen this type of smart metabolic training in action personally as Joy and I use various forms of it with fantastic results that show.

Studies show these efficient movements can burn up to 66% more calories, 900% more fat (that's NOT a misprint) and tone muscle at an 82% improved rate. Remember, harder isn't better, SMARTER is better.

Roy's Love: Kettle bells

If you can find a Kettle bell trainer nearby, you want to learn to work with kettle-bells; you can get results by just working with this Russian weight-fitness system for 4 minutes a day. For women, you develop a very strong core and gluteal muscles (think firm butt) and it is the most intense and satisfying training I know when you do it right.

Burning calories with everyday activities

When we look at exercise in general, it is important not just to stick to exercise in order loose weight and then spend the rest of the day watching TV or sitting behind a computer. The people who live the longest have an active life style, they mow the lawn and do a lot of walking; they only sit to rest or to have a conversation or eat! The high intensity exercise we propose here will make you younger and give you more energy, use that energy wisely!

The difference between a sitting and active lifestyle in calories burned is staggering.

You'll be happy to know that you can burn plenty of calories just by doing everyday activities.

"Research shows that people who are physically active during the day can burn an extra 300 calories per day," says Pete McCall, MS, an exercise physiologist with the American Council on Exercise. "Over 12 days, that can add up to an extra pound of weight loss," he says.

Burning calories: The "NEAT" way

McCall says that these extra 300 calories per day can come from what is called non-exercise activity thermogenesis, or NEAT, which accounts for the energy that you expend when you are not sleeping, eating, or doing structured physical activities like jogging or sports.

"NEAT" activities include things like walking or riding a bike for transportation, typing on the computer, working in the yard, and cleaning the house. Even fidgeting is considered a "NEAT" activity that can turn up your calorie-burning engine.

These activities help you burn calories by increasing your metabolic rate. This is why agricultural and manual workers tend to have higher metabolic rates than people who live more leisurely lifestyles. In fact, the calories burned through NEAT can differ by as much as 2,000 calories per day between two people who are similar in size.

We lived in Holland for a time and what you notice are the sheer amounts of bicycles in that country. Dutch people love to ride their bicycles to work and for shopping and continue doing that up into a ripe old age. They ride their cycles even in bad weather. Try cycling against the wind for an hour— that is a lot of NEAT activity. In the US driving a car is the favorite way of transportation and sometimes it is the only way to get to work. But if there is a chance to move your body on a bicycle even if it is just riding in nature, make it part of your leisure activities.

Burning calories: Totaling the burn

"NEAT" calories can really add up — and fast.

According to Kimberly Lummus, MS, RD, Texas Dietetic Association media representative and public relations coordinator for the Austin Dietetic Association in Austin, Texas, in 30 minutes a person who weighs 150 pounds can burn the following number of calories:

- Raking leaves = 147 calories
- Gardening or weeding = 153 calories
- Moving (packing and unpacking) = 191 calories
- Vacuuming = 119 calories
- Cleaning the house = 102 calories
- Playing with the kids (moderate activity level) = 136 calories
- Mowing the lawn = 205 calories
- Strolling = 103 calories
- Sitting and watching TV = 40 calories
- Biking to work (on a flat surface) = 220 calories

Burning calories: A little more every day

If you are trying to increase the number of calories you burn, make an effort to do more "spontaneous physical activities" throughout your day. The best way to do this is to reduce the time you spend sitting, while adding calorie-burning activities to your daily routine.

The following can increase your level of calorie burning throughout the day:

- Walk down the hall to see a colleague rather than making a phone call or sending e-mails
- Take the stairs instead of an elevator or escalator
- Clean your house instead of using a cleaning service
- Take your dog out for more frequent walks
- Ride your bike or walk to work rather than driving
- Park your car further away and walk a longer distance to your destination
- Make it a custom to go for a walk early morning or after dinner
- Plan hiking-weekends with friends

- Walk to a store if it is less than a 20 minute walk instead of driving
- If you have a 2 story house, walk the stairs up and down a few times during the day
- Take a 3 minute break every hour and do some knee bends (squats) or push ups or breathing/stretching exercises

Joy & Roy's big water tip #1

One great way to up your NEAT activity is to drink 3 liters of water a day, see Chapter 12; this has helped us tremendously to get up more from our chairs. Because of the sheer amount of water we have to go to the bathroom every half hour and we created 2 routines here. First is we go to the bathroom, which is furthest away from our desk; this forces us to walk a longer distance. The second routine is that we take a few minutes to stretch or do some squats or another short exercise. This helps the blood circulation, clear our minds and as has been proven scientifically to reset your brain so you actually function better! That is the extra benefit of drinking lots of water; it actually helps you lose weight in more ways than one!

Big tip #2

Consider wearing a pedometer to track the number of steps you take throughout the day. Once you have an idea of how many steps you take on average, set increasingly higher goals for yourself and find ways to take a few extra steps each day. Before you know it, you'll find yourself running up stairs, volunteering to sweep the porch, and finding reasons to walk to the store. The more you move, the more you'll want to move! There are some cool apps you can use to measure your daily activities; from "Jawbone Up", that also measure the efficiency of your sleep. You can now download on your computer your daily activity scores and work on increasing that every day.

Big tip #3

When you go shopping or to the office, consider parking further away. We normally search for the closest parking space, but what if you routinely park like a block away! That would add also to your NEAT activity and help you create an active lifestyle and of course taking the stairs when possible makes a big difference. See what other creative ways you can come up with to add miles or steps to your day so your body will become stronger and healthier.

5 reasons to walk more

We discussed that high intensity training is the best for losing weight, getting an after-burn and to activate more hormones that will rejuvenate your body.

That stands, the truth is that all activities where you activate your heart rate, stimulate your circulation will have an impact on your life. One of the reasons is that by doing something with your body you are stimulating your lymph circulation and you are burning calories, which is always good if you want to lose weight. This is where walking comes in as one of the preferred exercises after cycling to work and the grocery store if that is available.

Walking is a great, low-impact way to exercise. But, it also improves your mood and helps with your digestion. It is a great way to balance stress!

If you have a park close to where you live, you can drive there and go for your daily walk; if you live near hiking trails even better, make it a daily early morning or after work routine.

Taking a daily walk can help you stay in shape—and if you are obese or overweight, it's a low-impact way to ease into exercise; it also helps make your bones stronger.

5 more reasons for taking a walk

1. Walking Aids Digestion

According to research that appeared in *The New York Times*, a post-meal walk can aid digestion and control blood sugar levels. Alternatively, physically moving away from the dinner table eliminates the possibility of going back for seconds, thirds, or nineteenths. Over the years, researchers have found that a post-meal walk, as short as 15 minutes, can in fact help with digestion and improve blood sugar levels. In one study in 2008, German researchers looked at what happened when people ate a large meal and then consumed either an espresso or an alcoholic digestif — like brandy or flavored liqueur — or walked at a slow pace on a treadmill. Walking, they found, sped the rate at which food moved through the stomach. The beverages had no effect.

THE BOTTOM LINE Heading for a brief walk, instead of the couch, about 15 minutes after a meal may improve digestion and blood sugar control.

2. Walking is good for your bones

You won't bulk up in the same manner you would by performing load-bearing exercises like barbell squats or dead lifts, but walking still builds strength. Just a friendly warning: Avoid texting while walking. Texters are more accident prone because they have a less good balance and are less conscious of their environment.

3. Walking is low impact

If you are not ready for HIIT, then walking is a good place to start. When your goal is to lose weight aim to walk for a minimum of 20 minutes per day. If your still struggling with your nutrition and are addicted to carbs or other junk food or you are still at the beginning of the Sleep Your Fat Away program and you want consistent strong results, boost your walking time up to an hour per day. A good rate is 10,000 steps daily; get a pedometer so you can check it. IT-Walking: (Interval Training Walking) start with a brisk pace, so you really get your heart pumping and start with short sprints and recover and sprint again, get at least 6 sprints in your walking time where you either walk as fast you can or you actually run.

4. Walking can improve your mood

Sitting we know is bad when you have to do it for hours, scientific research shows that the longer we sit the shorter we live. Even when you exercise for an hour every day but you sit for prolonged time every day you shorten your life and you counteract your daily training! Especially when you sit all day under florescent lights, have to do a lot of computer work, dealing with lost of emails and boring meetings can be both frustrating and stressful. So, go regularly for a walk. Assuming you're not walking next to a freeway with traffic jam, the new stimuli and fresh air you encounter during a walk can help calm you down and give you more access to your creative brain. It helps to clear your head and can be a replacement for meditation, which we all need in today's stressful society. It's a fast way to boost mood…and a great way to detox both mentally and physically.

5. Walking cures laziness and is a great way to de-stress

There's no excuse not to take a walk. It is great when you are not ready to do the hardcore, intense exercise; by walking you are still being pro-active and it is a victory to accomplish this on a daily basis. If possible, add some stretching to your walking so you keep your body pliable and your joints and muscles flexible and in working order. Laziness kills, walking is a lifesaver.

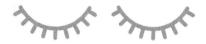

14

10 Tips To Accelerate Your Fat Loss

I f you're at all concerned about your health or your weight – whether you want to lose weight, gain health or maintain it – nutrition is paramount. We encourage you to start out with eating what you want when you begin with our program. It is vital that you break the cycle of starving and bingeing in order to be able to reconnect to your body's natural intelligence. You need to learn to hear what your body needs, to differentiate between emotional hunger and real hunger, and to take over the control of your emotional state. By following the simple guidelines we outlined in the chapter 11 "Stop Snacking and Start Eating" you will do just that.

Make a commitment and stick to it

Roy: I was unhappy with my appearance and extra weight (mostly around my belly and waistline), but I had the excuse that because I was travelling so much I could not follow a healthy lifestyle, exercise daily, and eat healthier foods. Part of me knew I was deceiving myself and yet it was a kind of comfort-zone. The underlying thought was that life was intense as it was and adding the regimen of exercising and watching what I eat was not going to make me happier. But there was always this conflict when I saw my belly in the mirror and it felt uncomfortable when friends made remarks about it. When one day my 3-year-old daughter pointed at my belly and asked if there was a baby inside, I knew the time had come to change. It was making the decision and standing up for who I was that started this whole idea going. That is when I decided that I would find the most successful person in weight loss and get help. Then the rest was easy. I did my research, heard of Sheila Granger and the journey began. After studying with her and many others to get the very best program together, Joy and I developed Sleep Your Fat Away. And I lost all my extra fat and was finally proud of my body again.

My journey began with making a commitment, making that one important decision to change. Now I am on cruise control, 40 pounds lighter and comfortable with my lifestyle of healthy foods, exercise and watching what I eat or snack. I follow the guidelines religiously and I make new decisions about what I put in my mouth! It all started with self-reflection on what I really wanted out of life: only when you have that clarity you can take off like a rocket!

Once you are on track and see how easy this is, you can take it a step further and reconsider your nutritional intake and lifestyle in general.

Taking part in a holistic program like ours give you the opportunity to take an honest look at the way you eat, live, and feel. This is why we asked you to answer some in depth questions at the beginning of the book, so you can get a detailed status quo.

The 2 components of successful, long-lasting weight loss

Understand that in order to stay healthy to an old age it is important to create a minimal delayed karmic effect of our lifestyle on our future!

Your health and body weight consists of two parts:

- Nutrition & lifestyle
- Mental & emotional state

Nutrition and lifestyle: Your diet accounts for about 80% of the health benefits reaped from a healthy lifestyle, with the remaining 20% stemming from exercise.

Eco-Foods are good for us (and the planet!)

A healthy diet will provide us with the foundation for longevity and is based on fresh whole, preferably organic foods, and foods that have been minimally processed.

What do you look for?

These are the signs of high-quality, health-promoting foods you'll want to look for when grocery shopping. If the food meets these criteria, it is most likely a wise choice, and would fall under the designation of "real food," which is the very foundation of good health and becoming slim and staying slim:

- It's grown without pesticides and chemical fertilizers (organic foods fit this description, but so do some non-organic foods)
- It's not genetically modified (the effects of the modified foods are untested for long term effects)
- It contains no added growth hormones, antibiotics, or other drugs (think of animals like cows and chickens)
- It does not contain any artificial ingredients, including chemical preservatives. (Processed foods with colorants and conservatives are not good for us)
- It is fresh (keep in mind that if you have to choose between wilted organic produce or fresh conventional produce, the latter may be the better option)
- It did not come from a concentrated animal feeding operation. These animals live disgraceful conditions. You don't want to have the stress hormones of the animals tainting your food!
- It is grown with the laws of nature in mind (meaning animals are fed their natural diets, not a mix of grains and animal by-products, and have free-range access to the outdoors and enough space to move).

- It is grown in a sustainable way (using minimal amounts of water, protecting the soil from burnout, and turning animal wastes into natural fertilizers instead of environmental pollutants)

A simple rule to also go by is: If you cannot pronounce the ingredients of a food product, don't eat it.

You have to understand that your food can either support you or cause problems for your body that will prevent a healthy life and a return to naturally slim body. As the great Anthony Robbins so rightly says: Your body has to either assimilate or eliminate what you are giving it!

You *can* be thin eating junk food but the long-term karmic effects are becoming sick and your body may become overburdened with toxins.

The program you are embarking on will help you to become a naturally thin person who is healthy and happy.

We are going for more than just losing weight, we want it all!

If you like that idea then you are on the right track, because this is consistent with the messages you will receive. You will notice that you prefer natural foods; you will start to invest in your health and your body. Processed foods and junk food will loose their appeal!

Does free will mean doing whatever you want?
The importance of your mental/emotional state

We have the free will to defy the natural programming of our body and its needs. You are not obliged to do anything; you don't have to eat healthy; you don't have to drink water. You can do what you want; that looks like free will, right?

But in reality it is not. There was a part of your mind that was programmed in a way when you had no free will: you have beliefs that are not yours; you were trained to eat in a certain way until you did not know another way. The choices you make are not completely your free will choices but the consequence of your subconscious programming. In other words many habits you developed over time were modeled by what you saw and what you were told. Your free will was taken from you when you were young: you had to do what your parents wanted you to do. You learned not to listen to your body but to follow certain rules, habits, and structure.

What we are doing is giving you back the power of your free will ...and you are the only one to decide what you want to choose.

You will learn again to *listen* to your body and to work *with* it so it becomes healthy, vital, slim and gets into optimal shape.

The programming we have developed for you, will remove the negative conditioning so you can listen to your body, break away from the old conditioning and discover what is best for you. Step by step you will discover what makes your body feel best; what gives you energy and what makes you healthy.

You become the captain of your ship once again.

Changing habits beautifully

Imagine this: You have made some big shifts and stuck to your new protocol for an entire week. Then you are invited out to a night out with your friends. You get delicious appetizers, fancy cocktails and maybe also due to the effect of a little too much alcohol, you have by this point have totally blown your new regime... so what's a little dessert to round it all off? Well, that logic has a name: the "what the hell" effect. Basically, when you cross a limit you've set for yourself, you lose control and just go all the way.

Researchers took this effect to the test and served participants a slice of pizza. Though the portions were equal, some slices were cut to *appear* larger or smaller than the others. Later, they asked participants to taste-test cookies, and allowed them to eat as many as they wanted. Dieters (or anyone watching their food intake) who *believed* they'd eaten a larger slice of pizza consumed more cookies than everyone else—50 percent more, in fact!

The effect on mood was even more interesting. People who tend to overeat felt worse if they ate the 'large' slice, while people who tend to restrict their diet felt *better*. This experiment shows us just how much our mind can trick us into post rationalizing virtually anything.

We are emotional...period

Extensive research on how people make decisions in sales, have proven time and time again that we are emotional beings, who make emotional choices, which we rationalize afterwards. And we are excellent in making an emotional decision sound rational!

Here's an interesting proof of this theory: A few years ago, neuroscientist Antonio Damasio made a ground breaking discovery. He studied people with damage in the part of the brain where emotions are generated. He found that they seemed normal, except that they were not able to feel emotions. But they all had something peculiar in common: they couldn't make decisions. They could describe what they should be doing in logical terms, yet they found it very difficult to make even simple decisions, such as what to eat. Many decisions have pros and cons on both sides—shall I have the chicken or the turkey? With no rational way to decide, these test subjects were unable to arrive at a decision. So at the point of decision, emotions are very important for choosing. In fact even with what we believe are logical decisions; the very point of choice is arguably always based on emotion.

What does this mean for our weight loss scenario?

If you are in an emotionally hyped or stressed state, you are not in the ideal state for making wise food choices. Think of the last times you ate unarguably unhealthy food and then remember what emotional state you were in at that time. Isn't it true that the pot of ice cream or bag of doughnuts is at it's most enticing when we are feeling upset, lonely, sad or stressed? So now think how liberating it is to have easy to use techniques that help you balance your emotions without having to resort to food. You wouldn't need to numb your emotions with sugar any more but could deal with them in a positive and powerful way.

Deprivation leads to binging

When you restrict your eating too much and feel deprived of the delicious foods you *really* want, you're more likely to swing to the other extreme. Remember the 3D trigger words! Diet, deprivation, and discipline. Your subconscious hears one of them and it goes into a tantrum… that's why dieters often gain the weight back, rather than keeping it off. You don't need to go into that destructive cycle because you are learning to deal with your emotions and have so many other helpers like the Virtual Gastric Band and Brain Training to support you.

Learn to replace one unhealthy habit with a new, healthier one.

Keep up your healthy habits by starting small and adding one change at a time. Incorporate healthy fats, fiber and lean proteins so you fill up on nutritious meals, but indulge in delicious treats in moderation. You'll be more satisfied (emotionally and physically) and be able to make a real life style change at the same time.

Habits: Most of the things you do every day are habits, and the wonderful thing about habits is that you don't have to think about them. You can plan your day while you drive your car to work without having to focus in detail on every step in the process.

The dark side of habits, though, comes when you try to change them. This is because habits are hard wired in your brain. Your brain has created synapses (a place in your nervous system where nerve cells join each other) to actually make your life easier. In order to change a habit, you need to change the synapses in your brain. And this is exactly where our tools come in: In Sleep your Fat Away! your brain is being trained to acquire new synaptic connections and create healthy habits night and day.

Here are 10 extra tips to help accelerate your fat loss

The hardest habits to break are the ones in which you used to do something that you want to stop doing – like not overeating or eating junk food.

The reason that these habits are so hard to break is that you typically try to replace doing *something* with doing *nothing*. The problem is that your brain is not designed to help you act. So, whenever you are in a situation where you used to perform the action you are trying to stop, your brain is going to suggest to you that you do it again. That means you have to exert willpower to stop yourself from doing the thing your brain is pushing you to do.

3 things you can do to help change your habits:

1) Replace doing something with doing something else.

Rather than trying to keep yourself from doing your habit all the time, try to create a new habit that operates in the same situation. If you are trying to stop biting your nails, buy a nail file and file them instead. Whenever you are in a situation where you used to bite your nails, train yourself to do something else. Smokers wanting to quit usually do best when they replace their (nasty) habit of smoking with a more health promoting one, such as exercising. One of our friends was a heavy smoker, when he decided to quit. He had not only smoked but also generally led a very unhealthy life eating junk food, drinking large quantities of alcohol and only moving from his desk to the refrigerator and then to bed. When he quit, he decided to go full blow: he started running, eating a healthy diet and within 6 months had not only stayed a happy non-smoker but was fit enough to run his first marathon. When we asked him why he had gone to such an extreme, he said: "Smoking took over such a big part of my life that without this habit, I felt kind of empty. So I decided to replace all the bad with a lot of good. And very quickly I got so fond of how good I felt; I amped up the levels of goodness even more… I have never felt any better!"

2) Tell a friend.

Your own motivation can break down easily, so enlist help. If for instance you're embarking on a radical change in lifestyle, find a friend who is willing to try it out too. Make it part of a team effort. This way you are not only committing (we feel much more obliged to stick to our promises if we make them in public), you are signing up to be accountable, and you have the added benefit of team motivation. When you feel like falling back into a bad habit, call up a your buddy and let her/him know. S/he can help talk you out of it.

3) Drink a glass of water and make yourself think.

Habits want to work on autopilot. So, when you're trying to change your behavior, set things up so that your autopilot doesn't work. Break the pattern by doing something that you wouldn't normally do in that moment, like drink a glass of water. You can make it even harder/more fun for yourself by drinking it standing on one leg or doing a push-up before you drink it.

If you are trying to lose weight, then rearrange the dishes and food storage in your kitchen. That way, none of the habitual ways that you ate at home before will work. You'll have to think about every step of the eating process, and that gives you a chance to add new behaviors.

Roy: I am quite an impatient person. I like seeing results and there is nothing I hate more than being stuck, like hitting a plateau and then feel like nothing is happening. This is why I am taking my weight loss to another level by finding ways to make the Sleep Your Fat Away even more effective. Here are some great ideas that I picked up from others who had great tips and I added a few of my own. Making these simple changes that either cut out or burn off extra calories will add up to weight loss over the course of a year. In the previous chapter we discussed HIIT and also the advantages of walking every day! That should be in your plan to have a healthy, firm slim body.

Watch out for the little things

One of the most important things I learned about being conscious about what I eat was keeping track of what goes in my mouth and then checking the results on the scale. So I know which indulgences will throw me off my path and what is simply not worth it. I used to routinely drink wine with my meals and discovered that it is not worth it unless there is a celebration of some sorts. By skipping or diminishing the amounts of the carbs like rice (my favorite), polenta (my other favorite), potatoes (love them), pasta (can you live without pasta?) my weight loss went much faster. If I really want some I would limit it instead of the portions I used to have, I would load up more on veggies, and salads. It is the little things that add up over time, the "little bit more" at the dinner buffet, going for the extra round of dessert, etc.

The little things in your favor

But what if you also knew about the little things you could do every day to increase your weight-loss success? Here are some extra tips for you that in the long term will make a big difference!

Here are the remaining 7 tips that will help you shed fat like melting snow on a hot day!

1. Snacks: enemies or friends?

YOU HAVE to change your snacking patterns (habits), especially if you work or live in an environment where there is abundance of snacking, like cookies in the office with the coffee or if you have a home with lots of 'goodies' for the kids.

First step: Elimination

If you know you can't resist brownies, cookies, or muffins, don't keep a mix in your pantry. Eliminate all temptations and replace with healthy choices as above

Second step: Anticipation

If you are going somewhere with friends and family and know you'll have a hard time controlling yourself, make a decision before you get there about what you will eat — and stick to it.

Create an abundance of healthy snacks like a fruit basket with apples, oranges, grapes, etc. Also think of bringing chopped up carrots, celery, etc instead of baked goodies. Make a plan for healthy snacks that combine a little bit of fat, **protein**, and crunch; such as apple slices smeared with peanut butter. Some walnuts, almonds and dried apple or mango can be healthy alternatives, if not overdone. If you are counting calories, doing the math may help: a pound of food has the equivalent of 3,500 calories, so if you can cut 100 calories out of your day, you will lose a pound in just over a month.

2. Banish all high-calorie condiments and sugars

A real no-no is sugar added to anything or getting drinks that have sugar in it (fructose, corn-syrup etc. are no-goes). So if you go to a coffee shop, avoid getting any added syrups. We are not fans of sweeteners but if you have to have something, try Splenda. Steevia or monk fruit are much better, but you will have to carry them with you, as most places don't serve them. In the long run it is better to wean yourself of the sweet taste, as this is still a ghost of the past (your childhood). Avoid mayonnaise: replace that with mustard on your burger or sandwich instead of mayonnaise, and always order your salad dressing on the side so that you can control the amount you eat.

3. Load up on veggies/salads

Your rule for life is that two thirds of your plate should be vegetables or salad. The one third can be split between protein or starchy carbohydrates (preferably one of the two). If you decide to get a second plate, which is unlikely when you follow the Sleep Your Fat Away program, it had better be all vegetables. People who routinely eat five or more servings of fruits and vegetables a day are much more successful with weight loss.

4. Ban fast food

A study of 1,713 adults who have been long term successful with weight loss demonstrated that people who eat at fast-food restaurants less than twice a week have greater success with their weight loss. If you do eat at a fast food restaurant than follow rule 3: load up on veggies and stop eating as soon as you feel satisfied. Just because it is a fast food restaurant does not mean you have to eat fast, if you eat consciously you will do fine.

5. Ban liquid calories

We have discussed this and you now know that water is your best friend and will help you lose weight. Most people understand that sugary sodas add calories; most people still believe that sweet tea and fruit juices are healthy. Big mistake, sweetened tea is no less calorie-dense than **soda**, and you are better off eating the fruit than drinking the juice.

6. Be accountable

The best way is to have a professional coach or if you cannot afford that, find a diet buddy you check in with or a support group. Keep a food diary; keeping track of your daily food choices takes only a few minutes, but can double your weight-loss success. (Roy) I have measured what effect certain foods had on my body and that way I have learnt what to avoid at all cost and what I can handle in what amounts.

7. Order smaller portions

Especially after you started the Sleep Your Fat Away program your brains still need time to break the old patterns that made you become overweight. So immediately start ordering smaller portions and ask the server to leave out the carbs for example and add extra veggies. Data suggests that people who order smaller portions or share a plate at restaurants are more successful with weight loss. So if available order the lunch portion, an appetizer, or a children's meal — or put up to half your meal into a doggy bag <u>before</u> you begin eating. If you used to order appetizers, skip that part and only go for the entrees, adapt the menu to your needs and give specific instructions to the waiter: no carbs, extra veggies (preferably without sauce), dressing on the side, etc.

8. Celebrate your success

To change your future, you need to believe you have it in you! You have to work on your beliefs and build up your self-confidence. People who believe they can succeed with weight loss actually do lose weight more successfully. How do you gain this confidence? Take a moment to pat yourself on the back when you make healthy choices and achieve your short-term goals.

These small changes, all of which are easily made, will quickly add up to more pounds lost over time.

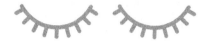

15

What Is In Your Sleep Your Fat Away Program?

When you buy our Sleep Your Fat Away package, you get everything you need to follow the program as a digital download. Once you have downloaded the files on to your computer, all you need to do is:

- Copy the audio files on to your mp3 player or Smartphone
- Read the guidelines
- Watch the short videos
- …And start!

In your package you receive

- 5 audio sessions plus 2 bonus sessions on the website
- Access to the videos explaining the techniques and strategies to combat stress, emotional hunger, cravings and our travel work out

- An e-booklet with the guidelines, background information and an overview of how to get the most out of your program.

We also created an extra audio (# 6: "Sleep Your Fat Away Maintenance Program"), which you will receive as a gift when you complete the program and send us your testimonial and a before and after picture. It is designed to help you stay on track and keep your desired weight for good. This audio is not included in the original download.

Audio #1
✓ **"Preparation for the Virtual Gastric Band"**
The first step to prepare your mind for losing weight! You listen to this session for 1 week and it prepares the mind to follow the instructions and gets you used to our voices. It also gets you ready for the installation of the Virtual Gastric Band, which will allow you to mentally shrink your stomach in size. Furthermore it adjusts your hunger to the level you need to lose weight.

Audio #2
✓ **"The Virtual Gastric Band Session"**
People often tell us how excited they are, when they are ready to hear this session. After listening to audio #1 for a week, this audio will take you on an imaginary visit to a Virtual Clinic and fit you with your new friend and helper: The Virtual Gastric Band. Experience shrinking your stomach to the size of an orange or larger golf ball; feel the immediate effects of being able to eat less effortlessly, be less hungry, have more energy and lose weight with mental power instead of will power.

Audio #3
✓ **8-hour Sleep Program**: "Sleep Your Fat Away"
This program consists of three (around 2 and half hour) sessions that are labeled 1, 2 and 3. Be sure to put them in that order. It is technically impossible to make an 8 hour MP#3 recording, so we had to break it down. This is the core of our unique program: lose weight while you sleep! This makes this program unique

and the most powerful weight loss system known to us. While you sleep you increase your metabolism to become an efficient fat-burner and dream about being and staying at your desired weight. Simply have this audio running in the background (no need for headphones!) and go to sleep. Imagine having your personal Sleep Your Fat Away therapist sit at your bedside and help you work on all the issues that are causing you to overeat or burn less fat. You will wake up each morning more energetic, happier and more positive.

Audio #4
✓ **High Speed Subliminals with Positive Affirmations**

You can listen to this audio just like having music in the background. Train your brain while you work. It will help you stay motivated and focused on eating healthily and moving your body more. This audio works directly on your subconscious mind without interference of your conscious mind. It's an easy and very powerful way of bypassing the critical mind. Your conscious mind will only hear gentle music, while your subconscious mind receives positive affirmations and empowering beliefs. Most people report how they feel more happy and uplifted when this is playing in the background. Put this audio on whenever you can while you are working or playing.

Audio #5
✓ **Reinforcement Pep Talk**

Whenever you have a setback or need a boost of energy or motivation, this short audio can lift your mood and helps you stay happy and positive. It's an ideal audio to listen to during the day and the perfect "excuse" to take a break or power nap with. Just by listening to it, you can—within minutes—transform a stressful situation into a benevolent one, just by training your brain to react in a more favorable and supportive way.

Audio #6 (not included in your download)
✓ **Sleep Your Fat Away Maintenance Program**

When you have lost all the fat you want to lose, this sleep program helps you maintain your desired weight. We have also added suggestions for the rejuvenation of your body, to support you in feeling healthier and biologically younger.

Guidelines
✓ The Guideline Booklet

This booklet explains the 6 guidelines for a life style make over to help you lose weight and achieve your goals with grace, ease, and joy. No diets, no pills, no willpower. You read it once and you have all the basics you need to change your life and leave the diet-struggles behind. Here we also share how to get the most out of your program and explain when to listen to which audio.

Videos
✓ Access to the videos: Emotional Balance Technique and Stress Point Hunger.

Learn in a short video how to transform all your emotions in less than 2 minutes and regain control. The second video explains the Stress Point Hunger, which helps you eat slower and more consciously. It is also a great Craving Buster.

No willpower needed—only mental power
As you can see this package is complete and unique, it contains all you need to lose weight and keep it off, forever. There is nothing else to buy or do. But let's be totally honest:

Important Note

As easy and effortless this program is to follow, you need to please make use of all parts! It is a revolutionary and intrinsically designed holistic approach that only requires you to follow some very simple guidelines. Please don't skip any part because you feel it's not important – trust us: every guideline and audio is essential for you to get the maximum effect!

Epilogue:
Are you serious about being slim and staying slim for the rest of your life?

Congratulations! You have read this book; thank you for bearing with us! Probably you have also read other books on weight loss, diets and lifestyle changes. We believe—based on our studies—we have created a method that works for anyone who is serious about losing weight and keeping it off. This is not for those die-hards who want a quick fix and then go back to their old lifestyles that created all the problems in the first place.

We are not from the diet industry selling pills and fancy low calorie diets; we are holistic life coaches, who have built a reputation for ourselves by getting results. We teach workshops all over the world to health professionals, holistic doctors, and the public.

We coach business people, athletes and celebrities and people who just want to be slimmer, healthier, happier, and more successful.

So if you are truly committed to getting results you have come to the right place.

Now it's your turn: Take action, go to our website and order the program, it is affordable and reliable: www.sleepyourfataway.com. As a side effect you will notice many good changes in your life. Our client's results show us that they become healthier, happier and have more fun in life.

We wish you all the best and are looking forward to your success stories!

With love,

Joy & Roy Martina

Resources
How We Can Help You

Webinars & Workshops

We conduct workshops and webinars all over the world on a wide array of subjects, all related to health, vitality, well being, personal development and success. You can inscribe for our free newsletter on www.christallin.com and www.joymartina. com. We also have a wide array of products on personal development. We have been leaders of this field in Europe for over 20 years.

Personal sessions through Skype

Ultimate results for Achievers and truly committed individuals

As our time is very limited, we can only take a few clients, mostly we work together on one client. We work mainly with Top executives and movers and shakers as they can make changes in their organization that can affect 1000's of people! See: www.theultimateresults.com for more information!

We feel very blessed to assist many high profile clients worldwide and see them blossom and thrive. Unfortunately we have not yet worked out how to multiply ourselves in a way that lets us help all those who contact us. So we sometimes have to turn down clients due to the lack of time. If destiny wants us to work with you, we will guide you for a minimum of 6 months to a year to make all the changes needed to guarantee your success. Send us a mail if you want to schedule a session: joeymartina@christallin.com or support@christallin.com. We will do our utmost to answer your mail as soon as we can.

Strategic Business Consulting

Another service we offer is Strategic Business Consulting.

We have clients worldwide. These are decision makers who want to take their companies to another level of success or profitability and are keen to do so in a karma positive way. We can advise on important decisions like hiring key-personnel, in which areas to invest more and find the parts of the company that are under-performing. Our clients get answers in a short time frame, as this is crucial when important decisions have to be taken. We can stand by and assist in negotiations and corporate meetings.

Addendum

Starting Your Journey

Step 1: Get a journal that is sacred to you

Step 2: Write the answers to these questions in your journal and review them every month!

Where are you now?

Here are some questions to help you reflect on where you are today: please write the answers down in your journal or on a blank piece of paper!

How much energy do you have throughout the day? When do you feel most tired?

What are your general stress levels like? Can you fall asleep easily at night?

Are you getting enough sleep? Do you wake up feeling refreshed or do you have to drag yourself out of bed in the morning?

Do you "need" a glass of wine or beer or do you just drink occasionally?

Do you drink enough water (2-3 quarts a day)? Do you drink diet drinks (where the sugar has been replaced with toxic substances like artificial sweeteners)?

162 | **SLEEP YOUR FAT AWAY**

Can you easily go without these for a week? Which sugary, caffeine infused drinks could you replace with water?

Are you happy with your level of fitness? Do you exercise? Can you climb the stairs; walk a good distance without getting out of breath? Can you play with your children without feeling like an old man/woman?

What are your biggest emotional triggers? How and when do you get most upset? What does someone have to do to get you stressed? When did you last lose your cool? And how did you react when it happened?

How do your emotions affect your eating habits? Do you eat more or less when you are stressed? What types of food do you chose when you are out of balance?

What are your craving foods? What are your snack culprits? What is the food you find hardest to stay away from?

Which food is a tradition in your family? What foods could your parents not do without?

Which foods do you remember being given as a treat as a child? What foods were "special" to you then?

Do you reward yourself with food and if so, what foods do you usually chose for this? How do you feel once you have indulged in these rewards?

How do you feel after eating in general? Do you feel energized and happy or more tired and guilty?

How often do you schedule time for yourself? How much time do you spend doing things for yourself? What do you do in your "me-time"?

How much time do you invest in your most important relationship (after yourself) – so with your partner, children and loved ones? How do you spend this time? Do you feel that you are spending quality time with them; does it feel emotionally rewarding to you?

Which relationships are creating most stress for you? What would it take for you to resolve this stress? What is holding you back from creating peace and/or speaking your truth?

What are your biggest fears? Where are you sabotaging yourself and procrastinating progress? What should you stop doing?

If you could chose for 5 miraculous changes in your life – what would they be? (Most people say more money and weight loss – so what are your other 3?)

And here some of our favorite life questions to take it a level deeper:

We learn from our mistakes, yet we're always so afraid to make one. Where is this true for you?

What risk would you take if you knew you could not fail?

What is your greatest strength? Have any of your recent actions demonstrated this strength?

What are the top five things you cherish in your life?

How old would you be if you didn't know how old you are?

When do you stop calculating risk and rewards, and just do it?

At what time in your recent past have you felt most passionate and alive?

What do you most connect with? Why?

What one piece of advice would you offer a newborn child?

Which is worse—failing or never trying?

Why do we do things we dislike and like the things we never seem to do?

What are you avoiding?

What is the one job/cause/activity that could get you out of bed happily for the rest of your life? Are you doing it now?

When it's all said and done, will you have said more than you've done?

What are you most grateful for?

What would you say is one thing you'd like to change in the world?

Do you find yourself influencing your world, or it influencing you?

Are you doing what you believe in or settling for what you're doing?

What are you committed to?

Which worries you more – doing things right or doing the right things?

If joy became the national currency, what kind of work would make you wealthy?

Have you been the kind of friend you'd want as one?

Do any of the things that used to upset you a few years ago matter at all today? What's changed?

Would you rather have less work to do or more work you enjoy doing?

What permission do you need/want to move forward?

Really, what do you have to lose if you go for it?

How different would your life be if there weren't any criticism in the world?

We're always making choices. Are you choosing for your story or for someone else's?

(By Blake Alexander Hammerton)

Write down the answers to these questions on a sheet of paper or in your weight loss journal. Don't judge or beat yourself up about how it is for you now. This exercise is to help you assess your status quo and more importantly help you define your future goals.

Setting your new goals

Now comes the fun part! Take another sheet of paper and write down 101 goals you want to achieve. Be as precise as possible. Be courageous! Consider all parts of your life. What do you want to achieve in this life, what do you want to have done before you leave Earth? After writing down the ones that come to mind easily like a new house, car, losing weight etc, you will be surprised what comes up!

In his national best selling book "The Success Principles" Jack Canfield suggest the wonderful idea of writing a Goals Book. Buy a journal or scrapbook and create a separate page for each one of your goals. Have fun illustrating each page: cut out images from magazines, use photographs, make it a visual feast! According to the Law of Attraction, your Goal Book (together with your body vision board) becomes script for your subconscious mind and the Universe to follow.

When writing your goals, pay attention to the way you specify them. You are not just writing down your wishes – you want crystal clear in your order to the Universe! So instead of writing: "I want to get fit," write something like: "I want to run a mile in 10 minutes by xxx (select a date)." Also make sure you set some goals that stretch you – you want to make the achievement of your goals part of your growth and development process. It's a good idea to define a few goals that make you feel slightly uncomfortable; goals that require you to learn new skills and go outside of your comfort zone.

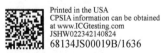
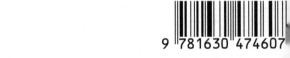